Pocket Guide to
Psychiatric Nursing

Pocket Guide to Psychiatric Nursing

Gail Wiscarz Stuart, PhD, RN, CS, FAAN

Center for Health Care Research
Professor, Colleges of Nursing and Medicine
Department of Psychiatry and Behavioral Sciences
Medical University of South Carolina
Charleston, South Carolina

Michele Teresa Laraia, PhD, RN, CS

Assistant Professor
Colleges of Medicine and Nursing
Department of Psychiatry and Behavioral Sciences
Medical University of South Carolina
Charleston, South Carolina

Fourth Edition

with illustrations

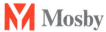 Mosby

A *Harcourt Health Sciences Company*
St. Louis   Philadelphia   London   Sydney   Toronto

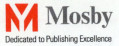
Mosby
Dedicated to Publishing Excellence

Vice President and Publisher: Nancy L. Coon
Editor: Jeff Burnham
Associate Developmental Editor: Jeff Downing
Project Manager: Gayle May Morris
Manufacturing Manager: Betty Mueller

Printed in the United States of America

Mosby Inc.
11830 Westline Industrial Drive
St. Louis, Missouri 63146

0-8151-2602-6

00 01 / 9 8 7 6 5 4 3 2

Contributors

SANDRA E. BENTER, DNSc, RN, CS
Psychotherapist and Consultant
Boca Raton, Forida

CAROLYN E. COCHRANE, PhD, RN, CS
Assistant Professor, Colleges of Medicine and Nursing
Associate Clinical Director, Eating Disorders Program
Department of Psychiatry and Behavioral Sciences
College of Nursing
Medical University of South Carolina
Charleston, South Carolina

LINDA V. JEFFERSON, PhD, RN, CS, CD
Research Manager
National Institute of Drug Abuse
Baltimore, Maryland

MARY D. MOLLER, MSN, ARNP, CS
Executive Director
The Center for Patient and Family Mental Health Education
Nine Mile Falls, Washington

MILLENE FREEMAN MURPHY, PhD, APRN
Associate Professor
College of Nursing
Brigham Young University
Provo, Utah

LINDA D. OAKLEY, PhD, RN
Assistant Professor
School of Nursing
University of Wisconsin–Madison;
Clinical Specialist in Adult Psychiatric and Mental Health Nursing
Madison, Wisconsin

CAROL K. PERLIN, MS, RN, CS
Director, Division of Patient Access and Emergency Services
Sheppard Pratt Health System
Baltimore, Maryland

SUSAN G. POORMAN, PhD, RN, CS
Associate Professor
Department of Nursing
Community College of Allegheny County-Boyce Campus
Pittsburgh, Pennsylvania

SANDRA J. SUNDEEN, MS, RN, CNAA
Chief, Division of Human Resource Development
Mental Hygiene Administration
Maryland Department of Health and Mental Hygiene
Adjunct Assistant Professor, School of Nursing
University of Maryland
Baltimore, Maryland

About the Authors

Dr. Gail Stuart is a tenured professor in the College of Nursing and a professor in the College of Medicine in the Department of Psychiatry and Behavioral Sciences at the Medical University of South Carolina. She received her BSN from Georgetown University, her MS in psychiatric nursing from the University of Maryland, and her PhD in Behavioral Sciences from Johns Hopkins University, School of Hygiene and Public Health. She is an American Nurses Association Certified Specialist in psychiatric and mental health nursing, a fellow in the American Academy of Nursing, a member of the American College of Mental Health Administrators, and a former president of the American Psychiatric Nurses Association.

Her current position at the Medical University of South Carolina is with the Center for Health Care Research, where Dr. Stuart works as a member of an interdisciplinary research team focusing on issues of access, resource utilization, and health-care delivery systems. She most recently was Administrator and Chief Executive Officer of the Institute of Psychiatry at the Medical University, where she was responsible for all clinical, fiscal, and human operations across the continuum of psychiatric care. Dr. Stuart has taught in undergraduate, graduate, and doctoral programs in nursing and is also active in clinical practice in the Department of Psychiatry. She serves on numerous academic, pharmaceutical, and governmental boards and represents nursing on a variety of National Institute of Mental Health policy and research panels. She is a strong advocate for the specialty and is in great demand to speak and consult throughout the United States and Canada. Dr. Stuart is a prolific writer and has numerous publications of articles, textbooks, and media productions. She has received many awards, including the American Nurses' Association Distinguished Contribution to Psychiatric Nursing–Current Impact on Innovations in Health Care Delivery Systems and Health Policy Award. Dr. Stuart's clinical and research interests involve the study of depression, anxiety disorders, and mental health delivery systems.

Dr. Michele Laraia is an assistant professor in the Colleges of Medicine and Nursing, Department of Psychiatry and Behavioral Sciences, Medical University of South Carolina in Charleston. She received her BSN at D'Youville College in Buffalo, New York, her MSN in psychiatric–mental health nursing at the University of Virginia, and her PhD in public health at the University of South Carolina. She has more than 25 years of experience in the field, including teaching, conducting research, and treating patients with psychiatric disorders. Her particular areas of expertise include psychobiology and psychopharmacology, for which she has a national reputation in the field. She designed and taught an innovative psychopharmacology course addressing the needs of advanced practice registered nurses who wanted to obtain prescriptive authority. At the Medical University she has taught psychiatric–mental health nursing at the master's level and holds a joint faculty appointment in the College of Graduate Studies. She is also involved in informatics and has served in various positions that focus on electronic medical records, networking systems, and patient confidentiality.

Dr. Laraia presents at a variety of psychiatric nursing conferences across the United States and has published and produced teaching media for the psychiatric nursing specialty. Her clinical practice focuses on people with depression, panic disorder with agoraphobia, and other anxiety disorders. She conducts research in the fields of Alzheimer's disease, depression, and anxiety disorders; is an investigator on various psychopharmacological clinical trials; and has received the American Psychiatric Nurses Association Award for Excellence in Research. Most notably, Dr. Laraia chaired the American Nurses' Association Psychopharmacology Task Force for Psychiatric–Mental Health Nurses.

Preface

Knowledge explosion . . . technology implosion. Each day the world of psychiatric nursing is bursting outward and inward with new information. The need to keep current with these changes is growing, but it often seems that the time to do so is shrinking. This reality is the reason for the fourth edition of the *Pocket Guide to Psychiatric Nursing*. This new edition has sharpened its focus in presenting the most current, relevant, practical, and concise information about psychiatric nursing care. The compact format emphasizes the essence of psychiatric nursing care and makes this content easily accessible to the nurse in the practical setting. The pocket guide also serves as an abbreviated complement to the comprehensive text from which it is derived, *Principles and Practice of Psychiatric Nursing*. Thus the reader of this pocket guide can learn more in-depth information about any clinical aspect of psychiatric nursing care by accessing the larger textbook, and students can use the pocket guide as a review and synthesis of content presented in the larger text.

This fourth edition has updated content throughout, information about the latest psychotropic medications, and a new chapter on the environmental context of psychiatric nursing care, which reviews the impact of managed care on contemporary practice. This edition also includes a new feature at the end of each chapter called Your Internet Connection, which lists World Wide Web sites that can be accessed on the Internet related to the chapter's content. In this way readers can stay current with rapidly emerging developments in each clinical area. The pocket guide continues to focus on the essentials of psychiatric nursing and is organized around the nursing process, thus providing assistance with conceptualizing, planning, and documenting nursing care. Nursing treatment plan summaries are included to provide for the clinical application of the nursing process to specific nursing care problems. Both DSM-IV medical and NANDA nursing diagnoses are provided, enabling the nurse to maintain a nursing focus while understanding the relationship with a medical approach. Each clinical chapter also includes a patient or family education plan. Whenever possible, tables and boxes are used to present material.

This pocket guide is divided into two parts. Part I, Principles of Psychiatric Nursing Care, consists of Chapters 1 through 8. This unit is designed to focus on the basic concepts of psychiatric nursing regardless of the patient care need or the practice setting. Chapter 1 discusses roles and functions of psychiatric nurses. Chapter 2 presents aspects of the therapeutic nurse-patient relationship, while Chapter 3 presents models of psychiatric–mental health practice. Chapter 4 describes the biopsychosocial context, Chapter 5 the environmental context, and Chapter 6 the legal-ethical context of psychiatric nursing care. The unit concludes with a discussion of the new ANA standards of clinical practice in Chapter 7 and nursing's role throughout the continuum of psychiatric care in Chapter 8, including primary prevention, crisis resolution, and rehabilitation.

Part II, Applying Principles in Nursing Practice, comprises the major content of the book. Chapters 9 through 19 consider nursing approaches to patients with specific nursing care problems, including anxiety, psychophysiological illness, self-concept, disturbances of mood, self-destructive behavior, psychotic and personality disorders, impaired cognition, substance abuse, eating disorders, and variations in sexual responses. The concluding two chapters discuss two specific types of treatment: psychopharmacology and somatic therapies. These chapters are particularly useful to nurses working in settings that are shifting to a more biological focus on the treatment of mental illness, and they include many explanatory tables and charts.

Finally, we are delighted that so many of you have told us that this book is an invaluable resource to you. We remain committed to providing you with the information that you need to give the best care possible to the patients who depend on you. We dedicate this book to you and all our psychiatric nursing colleagues who are so often unrecognized. We know that without you the pain and suffering of mentally ill people would often go unalleviated. If we have helped you to provide better psychiatric nursing care, our work has indeed been worthwhile.

Gail Wiscarz Stuart
Michele Teresa Laraia

Contents

PRINCIPLES OF PSYCHIATRIC NURSING CARE

Roles and Functions of Psychiatric Nurses

1

Psychiatric Nursing Defined and Described

Psychiatric nursing is an interpersonal process that strives to promote and maintain patient behavior that contributes to integrated functioning. The patient or client system may be an individual, family, group, organization, or community. The American Nurses' Association (ANA)[1] defines psychiatric and mental health nursing as:

A specialized area of nursing practice employing theories of human behavior as its science and purposeful use of self as its art.

The contemporary practice of psychiatric nursing occurs within a social and environmental context. The professional psychiatric nursing role has grown in complexity from its original historical elements. It now includes the dimensions of clinical competence, patient-family advocacy, fiscal responsibility, interdisciplinary collaboration, social accountability, and legal-ethical parameters.

The Center for Mental Health Services officially recognizes psychiatric and mental health nursing as one of the five core mental health disciplines. The psychiatric nurse uses knowledge from the psychosocial and biophysical sciences and theories of personality and human behavior to derive a theoretical framework on which to base nursing practice.

Levels of Performance

The following four major factors help to determine the levels of function and types of activities engaged in by a psychiatric nurse:

1. The nurse practice act of one's state
2. The nurse's qualifications, including education, work experience, and certification status
3. The nurse's practice setting
4. The nurse's degree of personal competence and initiative

The following two levels of psychiatric–mental health clinical nursing practice have been identified:

1. *A psychiatric–mental health registered nurse* (RN) is a licensed RN who has a baccalaureate degree in nursing and who has demonstrated clinical skills in psychiatric–mental health nursing that exceed those of a new nurse in the field. Certification is the formal process that validates the nurse's area of clinical expertise. The letter "C" placed after the RN (i.e., RN, C) designates basic-level certification status. Many professional nurses who contribute to the care of psychiatric patients have diplomas or associate degrees, are entry-level RNs, or are new to the specialty. These nurses practice with psychiatric–mental health RNs and are responsible for adhering to the specialty practice standards designated by the profession.

2. *A psychiatric–mental health advanced practice registered nurse* (APRN) is a licensed RN who has a master's degree, at a minimum, and in-depth knowledge of psychiatric nursing theory, supervised clinical practice, and competence in advanced psychiatric nursing skills. Doctorally prepared psychiatric–mental health nurses in advanced practice have both a master's degree and a doctorate in nursing or a related field. The letters "CS" placed after the APRN (i.e., APRN, CS) designate that the nurse is a *certified specialist* in psychiatric–mental health nursing.

Levels of Prevention

Psychiatric nursing interventions further include three areas of activity: primary, secondary, and tertiary prevention, as follows:

1. *Primary prevention* is a community concept that involves lowering the incidence of illness in a community by altering the causative factors before they have an opportunity to do harm. Primary prevention precedes illness and is applied to a generally healthy population. It includes health promotion and illness prevention.

2. *Secondary prevention* involves reducing the prevalence of actual illness by early detection and treatment of health problems.
3. *Tertiary prevention* involves reducing the impairment or disability that results from illness.

Continuum of Care

Traditional settings for psychiatric nurses include psychiatric facilities, community mental health centers, psychiatric units in the general hospital, residential facilities, and private practice. With health-care reform, however, alternative treatment settings throughout the continuum of mental health care have emerged for psychiatric nurses. Specifically, hospitals are being transformed into integrated clinical systems that provide inpatient care, partial hospitalization or day treatment, residential care, home care, and outpatient or ambulatory care. Current community-based treatment settings have been expanded to include foster care or group homes, hospices, home health agencies, visiting nurse associations, emergency departments, shelters, nursing homes, primary care clinics, schools, prisons, industry, managed care facilities, and health maintenance organizations (HMOs).

Competent Caring

The three domains of contemporary psychiatric nursing practice are: (1) direct care, (2) communication, and (3) management activities. The teaching, coordinating, delegating, and collaborating functions of the nurse's role are expressed within these overlapping domains of practice.

The various activities of psychiatric nurses within each one of these three domains can be further delineated. Box 1-1 lists the range of specific nursing activities that a psychiatric nurse could perform in each area. Although not all nurses participate in all these activities, they do reflect the current nature and scope of competent caring by psychiatric nurses. In addition, psychiatric nurses are able to do the following:

- Make biopsychosocial health assessments that are culturally sensitive.
- Design and implement treatment plans for patients and families with complex health problems and comorbid conditions.
- Engage in case management activities, such as organizing,

Box 1-1 Psychiatric Nursing Activities

Direct Care Activities

Activity therapy
Advocacy
Aftercare follow-up
Behavioral treatments
Case consultation
Case management
Cognitive treatments
Community assessment
Community education
Compliance counseling
Crisis intervention
Discharge planning
Environmental change
Environmental safety
Family interventions
Group work
Health promotion
Health teaching
High-risk assessment
Holistic interventions
Home visits
Individual counseling
Informed consent acquisition
Intake screening and evaluation
Medication administration
Medication management
Mental health promotion
Mental illness prevention
Milieu therapy
Nutritional counseling
Parent education
Patient triage
Physical assessment
Physiological treatments
Play therapy
Prescription medication duties
Psychoeducation
Psychosocial assessment
Psychotherapy

Treatment team meetings
Verbal reports of care

Management Activities

Budgeting and resource allocation
Clinical supervision
Collaboration
Committee participation
Community action
Consultation liaison
Contract negotiation
Coordination of services
Delegation of assignments
Grant writing
Marketing and public relations
Mediation and conflict resolution
Mentorship
Needs assessment and forecasting
Organizational governance
Outcomes management

Rehabilitative counseling
Relapse prevention
Research implementation
Self-care activities
Social skills training
Social systems support
Somatic treatments
Stress management

Communication Activities

Clinical case conferences
Documentation of care
Forensic testimony
Interagency liaison
Peer review
Professional nurse networking
Report preparation
Staff meetings
Transcription of orders
Treatment plan development

Continued

Box 1-1   Psychiatric Nursing Activities—cont'd

Management Activities—cont'd

Performance evaluations
Policy and procedure development
Practice guidelines formulation
Professional presentations
Program evaluation
Program planning
Publications
Quality improvement activities

Recruitment and retention activities
Regulatory agency activities
Risk management
Software development
Staff scheduling
Staff and student education
Strategic planning
Unit governance
Utilization review

accessing, negotiating, coordinating, and integrating services and benefits for individuals and families.

- Provide a health-care map for individuals, families, and groups to guide them to community resources for mental health, including the most appropriate providers, agencies, technologies, and social systems.
- Promote and maintain mental health and manage the effects of mental illness through teaching and counseling.
- Provide care for physically ill patients with psychological problems and psychiatrically ill patients with physical problems.
- Manage and coordinate systems of care integrating the needs of patients, families, staff, and regulators.

Outcome Evaluation

Psychiatric nurses must be able to identify, describe, and measure the effect of the care they provide patients, families, and communities. *Outcomes* are those factors that affect the patient and family while they are involved in the health-care system, including health status, functional status, quality of life, presence or absence of illness, type of coping response, and satisfaction with treatment. Outcome evaluation can focus on a clinical condition, an intervention, or the caregiving process.

Critically evaluating the outcomes of psychiatric nursing activities is a task for every psychiatric nurse, regardless of role, qualifications, or practice setting. Psychiatric nurse clinicians, educators, administrators, and researchers all must assume responsibility for answering the question. What difference does psychiatric nursing care make?

your **INTERNET**
c o n n e c t i o n

American Psychiatric Nurses Association: http://www.apna.org
Canadian Federation of Mental Health Nurses: http://www.iciweb.com/cfmhn

Reference

1. American Nurses' Association: *Statement on psychiatric–mental health clinical nursing practice and standards of psychiatric–mental health clinical nursing practice,* Washington, DC, 1994, The Association.

Suggested readings

Billings C: Psychiatric–mental health nursing professional progress notes, *Arch Psychiatr Nurs* 7:174, 1993.

Cohen S, et al: Stages of nursing's political development: Where we've been and where we ought to go, *Nursing Outlook* 44:259, 1996.

Krauss J: *Health care reform: essential mental health services,* Washington, DC, 1993, American Nurses' Association.

Lanza M: Power and leadership in psychiatric nursing: Directions for the next century, Part I and II, *Perspectives in Psychiatric Care* 33:5, 1997.

McBride A: Psychiatric–mental health nursing in the twenty-first century. In McBride A, Austin J, editors: *Psychiatric–mental health nursing: integrating the behavioral and biological sciences,* Philadelphia, 1996, WB Saunders.

Merwin E, Mauck A: Psychiatric nursing outcome research: the state of the science, *Arch Psychiatr Nurs* 9:311, 1995.

Olson T: Fundamental and special: the dilemma of psychiatric–mental health nursing, *Arch Psychiatr Nurs* 10:3, 1996.

Pearson L: Annual update of how each state stands on legislative issues affecting advanced nursing practice, *Nurse Pract* 22:18, 1997.

Stuart G: An organizational strategy for empowering nursing, *Nurs Econ* 4:35, 1986.

Stuart G, Laraia M: *Principles and practice of psychiatric nursing,* ed 6, St Louis, 1998, Mosby.

Therapeutic Nurse-Patient Relationship

The therapeutic nurse-patient relationship is a mutual learning experience and a corrective emotional experience for the patient. In this relationship the nurse uses the self and specified clinical techniques in working with the patient to bring about insight and behavioral change.

Nature of the Relationship

The goals of a therapeutic relationship are directed toward the patient's growth and include the following:

1. Self-realization, self-acceptance, and increased self-respect
2. Clear sense of personal identity and improved personal integration
3. Ability to form intimate, interdependent, interpersonal relationships with a capacity to give and receive love
4. Improved functioning and increased ability to satisfy needs and achieve realistic personal goals

To achieve these goals, various aspects of the patient's life experiences are explored during the course of the relationship. The nurse allows for the patient's expression of perceptions, thoughts, and feelings and relates these to observed and reported actions. Areas of conflict and anxiety are clarified. It is also important for the nurse to identify and maximize the patient's ego strengths and to encourage socialization and family relatedness. Problems of communication are corrected and maladaptive behavior patterns modified as the patient tests out new patterns of behavior and more adaptive coping mechanisms. Figure 2-1 shows the elements that produce a therapeutic outcome.

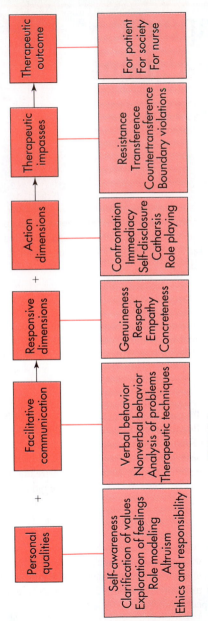

Figure 2-1

Elements affecting the nurse's ability to be therapeutic.

Therapeutic Use of Self

The principal helping tool that the psychiatric nurse can use in practice is the self. Thus self-analysis is an essential aspect of being able to provide therapeutic nursing care. Specific personal qualities needed by the nurse who wants to be therapeutic include the following:

1. Self-awareness
2. Clarification of values
3. Exploration of feelings
4. Ability to serve as role model
5. Altruistic motivations
6. Sense of ethics and responsibility

Phases of the Relationship

The four sequential phases of the nurse-patient relationship are (1) preinteraction phase, (2) introductory or orientation phase, (3) working phase, and (4) termination phase. Table 2-1 summarizes the nurse's tasks in each phase of the relationship process.

Facilitative Communication

Communication theory is relevant to psychiatric nursing practice for three major reasons. First, communication is the vehicle for establishing a therapeutic relationship because it involves conveying information and exchanging thoughts and feelings. Second, communication is the means by which people influence the behavior of others. Therefore communication is critical to the successful outcome of nursing intervention, because the nursing process is directed toward promoting adaptive behavioral change. Finally, communication is the relationship itself; without it, a therapeutic nurse-patient relationship is not possible.

Levels of Communication

Verbal communication occurs through the medium of words, spoken or written, and represents a small segment of total human communication. Validation of the meaning of verbal communication between the nurse and patient is essential.

   Nonverbal communication involves all five senses and includes everything that does not involve the written or spoken word. The five categories of nonverbal communication are as follows:

1. *Vocal cues* are paralinguistic or extraspeech noises and sounds.

Table 2-1   Nursing tasks in each phase of a therapeutic relationship

Phase	Task
Preinteraction	Explore own feelings, fantasies, and fears. Analyze own professional strengths and limitations. Gather data about patient when possible. Plan for first meeting with patient.
Introductory or orientation	Determine reason patient sought help. Establish trust, acceptance, and open communcation. Explore patient's thoughts, feelings, and actions. Identify patient's problems. Define goals with patient. Mutually formulate contract to include names, roles, responsibilities, expectations, purpose, meeting location, time of meetings, conditions for termination, and confidentiality.
Working	Explore relevant stressors. Promote patient's development of insight and use of constructive coping mechanisms. Discuss and overcome resistance behaviors.
Termination	Establish reality of separation. Review progress of therapy and attainment of goals. Mutually explore feelings of rejection, loss, sadness, and anger and related behaviors.

2. *Action cues* are all body movements, including facial expression and posture.
3. *Object cues* are a person's intentional and nonintentional use of objects, such as dress and possessions.
4. *Space* is the physical distance between two people.
5. *Touch* is physical contact between two people and is the most personal nonverbal communication.

The Communication Process

Human communication is a dynamic process that is influenced by the psychological and physiological conditions of the participants.

The structural model of communication identifies the following five functional components:

1. *Sender*—originator of the message
2. *Message*—unit of information transmitted from the sender to the receiver
3. *Receiver*—perceiver of the message, whose behavior is influenced by the message
4. *Feedback*—response of the receiver to the sender
5. *Context*—setting in which the communication takes place

If a nurse evaluates the communication process with regard to these five structural elements, specific problems or potential errors can be identified.

Therapeutic Communication Techniques

Two requirements of effective communication are: (1) that it be aimed at preserving the self-respect of both the nurse and the patient and (2) that the communication of acceptance and understanding precedes any suggestions of information or more specific information. Various methods exist for recording nurse-patient communications, including videotape, sound recording, and verbatim, outline, and postinteraction notes. Table 2-2 identifies various therapeutic communication techniques with definitions, examples, therapeutic value, and nontherapeutic threats.

Dimensions of the Relationship

The nurse must acquire certain skills or qualities to initiate and continue a therapeutic relationship. These skills incorporate verbal and nonverbal behavior and the attitudes and feelings behind the nurse's communication. They are broadly divided into responsive and action dimensions, as follows:

1. *Responsive dimensions* include genuineness, respect, empathic understanding, and concreteness. They are crucial in the orientation phase of the relationship to establish trust and open communication. They continue to be useful throughout the working and termination phases and allow the patient to achieve insight.
2. *Action-oriented dimensions* include confrontation, immediacy, nurse self-disclosure, emotional catharsis, and role playing. They must be implemented in the context of warmth, acceptance, and understanding established by the responsive dimensions. They help the therapeutic relation-

Table 2-2   Therapeutic communication techniques

Technique	Definition	Example	Therapeutic Value	Nontherapeutic Threat
Listening	Active process of receiving information and examining one's reaction to messages received	Maintaining eye contact and receptive nonverbal communication	Nonverbally communicates to nurse's interest and acceptance to patient	Failure to listen
Broad openings	Encouraging patient to select topic for discussion	"What are you thinking about?"	Indicates acceptance by nurse and value of patient's initiative	Domination of interaction by nurse; rejection of responses
Restating	Repeating to patient the main thought patient has expressed	"You say that your mother left you when you were 5 years old."	Indicates nurse is listening and validates, reinforces, or highlights something patient has said	Lack of validation of nurse's interpretation of message; being judgmental; reassuring; defending

Clarification	Attempting to put into words vague ideas or unclear thoughts of patient, or asking patient to explain what is meant	"I'm not sure what you mean. Could you tell me that again?"	Helps to clarify patient's feelings, ideas, and perceptions, and provides explicit correlation between them and patient's actions	Failure to probe; assumed understanding
Reflection	Directing patient's ideas, feelings, questions, and content back to patient	"You're feeling tense and anxious, and it's related to a conversation you had with your mother last night?"	Validates nurse's understanding of what patient is saying and indicates empathy, interest, and respect for patient	Stereotyping patient's responses; inappropriate timing and depth of feeling; inappropriate response to patient's cultural experience and educational level
Focusing	Questions or statements that help patient expand on topic of importance	"I think we should talk more about your relationship with your father."	Allows patient to discuss central issues and keeps communication goal directed	Allowing abstractions and generalization; changing topics

Continued

Table 2-2 Therapeutic communication techniques—cont'd

Technique	Definition	Example	Therapeutic Value	Nontherapeutic Threat
Sharing perceptions	Asking patient to verify nurse's understanding of what patient is thinking or feeling	"You're smiling, but I sense that you're really very angry with me."	Conveys nurse's understanding and may clear up confusion	Challenging patient; accepting literal responses; reassuring; testing; defending
Identifying themes	Underlying issues or problems that emerge repeatedly	"I've noticed that in all the relationships you describe, you've been hurt by the man. Do you think this is an underlying issue?"	Allows nurse to best promote patient's exploration and understanding of important problems	Giving advice; reassuring; disapproving
Silence	Lack of verbal communication for therapeutic reason	Sitting with patient and nonverbally communicating interest and involvement	Allows patient time to think and gain insights, slows pace of interaction, and encourages patient to initiate conversation while nurse conveys support, understanding, and acceptance	Questioning patient; asking for "why" responses; failure to break nontherapeutic silence

| Humor | Discharge of energy through comic enjoyment of the imperfect | "That gives a whole new meaning to the word 'nervous,'" said with shared kidding. | Can promote insight by making conscious repressed topics; can resolve paradoxes, temper aggression, and reveal new options; is a socially acceptable form of sublimation | Indiscriminate use; belittling patient; screen to avoid nontherapeutic initimacy |

ship progress by identifying obstacles to the patient's growth and by underscoring the need for not only internal understanding or insight, but also external action and behavioral change.

Table 2-3 summarizes the responsive and action dimensions for therapeutic nurse-patient relationships.

Therapeutic Impasses

Therapeutic impasses, or blocks in the progress of the nurse-patient relationship, are of three primary types: resistance, transference, and countertransference. They arise from a variety of reasons and may take many different forms, but they all create stalls in the therapeutic relationship. Therefore the nurse should deal with them as soon as possible. These impasses provoke intense feelings in both the nurse and the patient that may range from anxiety and apprehension to frustration, love, or intense anger.

Resistance

Resistance is the patient's attempt to remain unaware of anxiety-producing aspects within the self. It is a natural reluctance to or learned avoidance of verbalizing or even experiencing the troubled aspects of oneself. Ambivalent attitudes toward self-exploration, in which the patient both appreciates and avoids anxiety-producing experiences, are a normal part of the therapeutic process. A primary resistance is often the result of the patient's unwillingness to change when the need for change is recognized. Resistance behaviors are usually displayed by patients during the working phase of the relationship, because it contains most of the problem-solving process. Box 2-1 lists forms of resistance displayed by patients.

Transference

Transference is an unconscious response in which the patient experiences feelings and attitudes toward the nurse that were originally associated with significant figures in the patient's early life. The term refers to a group of reactions that attempt to reduce or alleviate anxiety. The outstanding traits defining transference are the inappropriateness of the patient's response in terms of intensity and the maladaptive use of the defense mechanism of displacement.

Table 2-3   Responsive and action dimensions for therapeutic nurse-patient relationships

Dimension	Characteristics
Responsive Dimensions	
Genuineness	Implies that nurse is an open person who is self-congruent, authentic, and accessible
Respect	Suggests that patient is regarded as a person of worth who is valued and accepted without qualification
Empathic understanding	Viewing patient's world from patient's internal frame of reference, with sensitivity to patient's current feelings and with verbal ability to communicate this understanding in language appropriate to patient
Concreteness	Involves use of specific terminology rather than abstractions in discussion of patient's feelings, experiences, and behavior
Action Dimensions	
Confrontation	Nurse's expression of perceived discrepancies in patient's behavior to expand patient's self-awareness
Immediacy	Occurs when current nurse-patient interaction in relationship is used to learn about patient's functioning in other interpersonal relationships
Nurse self-disclosure	Evident when nurse reveals information about self and own ideas, values, feelings, and attitudes to facilitate patient's cooperation, learning, catharsis, or support
Emotional catharsis	Patient encouraged to talk about most bothersome aspects of life for therapeutic effect
Role playing	Acting out a particular situation to increase patient's insight into human relations and deepen patient's ability to see a situation from another point of view; also allows patient to experiment with new behavior in a safe environment

Box 2-1   Forms of Resistance

- Suppression and repression of pertinent information
- Intensification of symptoms
- Self-devaluation and hopeless outlook on the future
- Forced flight into health, in which patient experiences a sudden but short-lived recovery
- Intellectual inhibitions, which may be evident when patients say they have nothing on their mind or are unable to think about their problems; break appointments or arrive late for sessions; or are forgetful, silent, or sleepy
- Acting-out or irrational behavior
- Superficial talk
- Intellectual insight, in which patient verbalizes self-understanding with correct use of terminology yet continues maladaptive behavior, or use of the defense of intellectualization when no insight exists
- Contempt for normality, which is evident when patient has developed insight but refuses to assume responsibility for change on the grounds that normality is not so appealing
- Transference reactions

Transference reactions are harmful to the therapeutic process only if they remain ignored and unexamined by the nurse. The two main types are hostile and dependent reactions.

Countertransference

Countertransference is a therapeutic impasse created by the nurse, not the patient. It refers to a specific emotional response by the nurse to the patient that is inappropriate to the content and context of the therapeutic relationship or inappropriate in its emotional intensity. Countertransference is transference applied to the nurse. The nurse's responses are not justified by reality but rather reflect previous conflicts experienced with issues such as authority, gender assertiveness, and independence.

Countertransference reactions are usually one of three types: reactions of intense love or caring, reactions of intense

Box 2-2   Forms of Countertransference Displayed by Nurses

- Difficulty empathizing with patient in certain problem areas
- Feeling depressed during or after session
- Carelessness about implementing contract, such as being late or running overtime
- Drowsiness during sessions
- Feeling angry or impatient because of patient's unwillingness to change
- Encouraging patient's dependency, praise, or affection
- Arguing with patient or tendency to "push" patient before ready
- Trying to help patient in matters not related to identified nursing goals
- Personal or social involvement with patient
- Dreaming about or preoccupation with patient
- Sexual or aggressive fantasies toward patient
- Recurrent anxiety, unease, or guilt related to patient
- Tendency to focus on only one aspect of information presented by patient or to view it only one way
- Need to defend nursing interventions with patient to others

hostility or hatred, and reactions of intense anxiety, often in response to a patient's resistance. Box 2-2 presents some forms of countertransference.

Boundary Violations

Boundary violations occur when a nurse goes outside the boundaries of the therapeutic relationship and establishes a social, economic, or personal relationship with a patient. As a general rule, whenever the nurse is doing or thinking of doing something special, different, or unusual for a patient, a boundary violation usually is involved. Box 2-3 lists examples of possible boundary violations.

Box 2-3 Possible Boundary Violations Related to Psychiatric Nurses

- Patient takes nurse out to lunch or dinner.
- Professional relationship turns into social relationship.
- Nurse attends a party at patient's invitation.
- Nurse regularly reveals personal information to patient.
- Patient introduces nurse to family members, such as a son or daughter, for the purpose of a social relationship.
- Nurse accepts free gifts from patient's business.
- Nurse agrees to meet patient for treatment outside the usual setting without therapeutic justification.
- Nurse attends social functions of patient.
- Patient gives nurse an expensive gift.
- Nurse routinely hugs or has physical contact with patient.
- Nurse does business with or purchases services from patient.

Overcoming Therapeutic Impasses

To overcome therapeutic impasses, the nurse must be prepared to be exposed to powerful emotional feelings within the context of the nurse-patient relationship. Initially the nurse must have knowledge of the impasses and recognize behaviors that indicate their existence. Then the nurse can clarify and reflect on feeling and content to focus more objectively on what is happening.

The reasons behind the behavior are explored, and either the patient (for resistance and transference reactions) or the nurse (for countertransference reactions and boundary violations) accepts responsibility for the impasse and its negative impact on the therapeutic process. Finally, the goals of the relationship and the areas of the patient's needs and problems are reviewed. This should help the nurse reestablish a therapeutic alliance consistent with the process of the nurse-patient relationship.

your **INTERNET**

c o n n e c t i o n

National Institute of Mental Health: http://www.nimh.nih.gov

Internet Mental Health: http://www.mentalhealth.com

Suggested readings

Albert G: What are the characteristics of effective psychotherapists? The experts speak, *J Pract Psychiatry Behav Health* 3:35, 1997.

Carkhoff R: *Helping and human relations,* vols 1 and 2, New York, 1969, Holt, Rinehart & Winston.

Epstein R: *Keeping boundaries: maintaining safety and integrity in the psychotherapeutic process,* Washington, DC, 1994, American Psychiatric Press.

Forchuk C: Development of nurse-client relationships: what helps? *J Am Psychiatr Nurs Assoc* 1:146, 1995.

Krupnick J et al: The role of the therapeutic alliance in psychotherapy and pharmacotherapy outcome: findings from the National Institute of Mental Health Treatment of Depression Collaborative Research Program, *J Consult Clin Psychol* 64:532, 1996.

Miles M: The evolution of countertransference and its application to nursing, *Perspect Psychiatr Care* 29:13, 1993.

Montgomery C: *Healing through communication: the practice of caring,* Newbury Park, Calif, 1993, Sage.

Muller A, Poggenpoel M: Patients' internal world experiences of interacting with psychiatric nurses, *Arch Psychiatr Nurs* 10:143, 1996.

Nichols M: *The lost art of listening,* New York, 1995, Guilford.

Pilette P, Bereck C, Archber L: Therapeutic management of helping boundaries, *J Psychosoc Nurs* 33:40, 1995.

Stuart G, Laraia M: *Principles and practice of psychiatric nursing,* ed 6, St Louis, 1998, Mosby.

Sundeen S et al: *Nurse-client interaction: implementing the nursing process,* ed 6, St Louis, 1998, Mosby.

Models of Psychiatric–Mental Health Practice

3

Defining Mental Health and Mental Illness

Health-illness and adaptation-maladaptation are distinct concepts. Each exists on a separate continuum. The health-illness continuum derives from a medical world view. The adaptation-maladaptation continuum derives from a nursing world view. Thus a person who has a medically diagnosed illness, whether physical or psychiatric, can be adapting well to it. In contrast, a person who does not have a medically diagnosed illness may have many maladaptive coping responses. These two continuums reflect how nursing and medical models of practice complement each other.

Mental Health

The following have been identified as criteria of mental health:
1. Positive attitudes toward self
2. Growth, development, and self-actualization
3. Integration and emotional responsiveness
4. Autonomy and self-determination
5. Accurate reality perception
6. Environmental mastery and social competence

Mental Illness

One's definition of mental illness is derived from what one believes to be the causative factors. The following hypotheses have been proposed to influence the occurrence of mental illness:
1. *Biological hypothesis* proposes anatomical and physiological dysfunctions.

2. *Learning hypothesis* proposes maladaptive learned behavioral patterns.
3. *Cognitive hypothesis* proposes inaccuracies or deficits in knowledge or awareness.
4. *Psychodynamic hypothesis* proposes intrapsychic conflicts and developmental deficits.
5. *Environmental hypothesis* proposes stressors and aversive environmental responses.

Box 3-1 presents key facts about mental illness.

Box 3-1   Key Facts About Mental Illness

Extent and Severity of the Problem

- The full spectrum of mental disorders affects 22% of the adult population in a given year. This figure refers to *all* mental disorders and is comparable to rates for physical disorders when similarly broadly defined (e.g., respiratory disorders affect 50% of adults; cardiovascular diseases, 20%).
- Severe mental disorders (i.e., schizophrenia, manic-depressive illness, and severe forms of depression, panic disorder, and obsessive-compulsive disorder) affect 2.8% of the adult population (approximately 5 million people) and account for 25% of all Federal disability payments.
- At least 7.5 million children in the United States under 18 years of age have a mental health problem severe enough to require treatment.
- Approximately 18 million persons in the United States 18 years of age and older experience problems as a result of alcohol use; 10.6 million of these have alcoholism.
- Most alcoholic persons improve through treatment, and evidence suggests that alcoholism treatment is effective in containing costs throughout the health-care system and increasing worker productivity.
- An estimated 23 million people in the United States currently use illicit drugs.

Continued

Box 3-1   Key Facts About Mental Illness—cont'd

Treatment Efficacy

- How *effective* are treatments for severe mental disorders compared with treatments for physical illness?

Disorder	Treatment Success Rate
Panic	80%
Bipolar	80%
Major depression	65%
Schizophrenia	60%
Obsessive-compulsive	60%
Cardiovascular treatments	
Atherectomy	52%
Angioplasty	41%

From National Advisory Mental Health Council: Am J Psychiatry *150:1447, 1993.*

Conceptual Models of Practice

Many mental health professionals practice within the framework of a conceptual model. A *model* is a means of organizing a complex body of knowledge, such as concepts related to human behavior. Using a model helps a clinician to develop a sound basis for assessment and intervention, as well as a way to evaluate the effectiveness of treatment. A number of conceptual models are used in psychiatric practice. Table 3-1 presents these models and associated theorists, their view of behavioral deviations, the therapeutic process, and the roles of the patient and therapist.

The Stuart Stress Adaptation Model of Psychiatric Nursing Care

Psychiatric nurses can practice more effectively if their actions are based on a model that recognizes the presence of health or illness as an outcome of multiple characteristics of a person interacting with environmental factors. The Stuart Stress Adaptation Model of psychiatric nursing care integrates the biological, psychological, sociocultural, environmental, and legal-ethical aspects of nursing into a unified framework for practice

Text continued on p. 35

Table 3-1 Models of psychiatric mental health practice

Model (Major Theorists)	View of Behavioral Deviation	Therapeutic Process	Roles of Patient and Therapist
Psychoanalytical (S. Freud, Erikson, Klein, Horney, Fromm-Reichmann, Menninger)	Behavior is based on early development and inadequate resolution of developmental conflicts. Ego defenses unable to control anxiety. Symptoms result as effort to deal with anxiety and are related to unresolved conflicts.	Psychoanalysis uses techniques of free association and dream analysis. It interprets behavior, uses transference to revise earlier traumatic experiences, and identifies problem areas through interpretation of patient's resistances.	Patient verbalizes all thoughts and dreams and considers therapist's interpretations. Therapist remains remote to encourage development of transference and interprets patient's thoughts and dreams in terms of conflicts, transference, and resistance.

Continued

Table 3-1   Models of psychiatric mental health practice—cont'd

Model (Major Theorists)	View of Behavioral Deviation	Therapeutic Process	Roles of Patient and Therapist
Interpersonal (Sullivan, Peplau)	Anxiety arises and is experienced interpersonally. The basic fear is fear of rejection. Person needs security and satisfaction that result from positive interpersonal relationships.	Relationship between therapist and patient builds feeling of security. Therapist helps patient experience trusting relationship and gain interpersonal satisfaction. Patient then assisted to develop close relationships outside therapy situation.	Patient shares anxieties and feelings with therapist. Therapist develops close relationship with patient; uses empathy to perceive patient's feelings and uses relationship as a corrective interpersonal experience.

Social (Szasz, Caplan)	Social and environmental factors create stress, which causes anxiety, resulting in symptom formation. Unacceptable (deviant) behavior is socially defined and meets needs of social system.	Patient helped to deal with social system. Crisis intervention may be used. Environmental manipulation and enlistment of special supports are also employed. Peer support is encouraged.	Patient actively presents problem to therapist and works with therapist toward resolution. Community resources are used. Therapist explores patient's social system and helps patient use resources available or create new resources.
Existential (Peris, Glasser, Ellis, Rogers, Frankl)	Life is meaningful when person can fully experience and accept the self. Behavioral deviation occurs when individual is thwarted in the effort to find and accept self. The self can be experienced through authentic relationships with other people.	Person aided to experience authenticity in relationships. Therapy is frequently conducted in groups. Patient is encouraged to explore and to accept self and helped to assume control of behavior.	Patient assumes responsibility for behavior and participates in meaningful experiences to learn about real self. Therapist helps patient to recognize value of self. Therapist clarifies realities of situation and introduces patient to genuine feelings and expanded awareness.

Continued

Table 3-1   Models of psychiatric mental health practice—cont'd

Model (Major Theorists)	View of Behavioral Deviation	Therapeutic Process	Roles of Patient and Therapist
Supportive (Werman, Rockland)	Problems are a result of biopsychosocial factors. Emphasis on current maladaptive coping responses.	Reality testing and self-esteem enhancing measures. Social supports are enlisted and adaptive coping responses reinforced.	Patient actively involved in treatment. Therapist is warm and empathic and allies with patient.
Communication (Berne, Watzlawick)	Behavioral disruptions occur when messages are not clearly communicated. Language can be used to distort meaning. Messages may be transmitted simultaneously at several levels. Verbal and nonverbal messages may lack congruence.	Communication patterns analyzed and feedback given to clarify problem areas. Transactional analysis focuses on games and learning to communicate directly without game playing.	Patient examines communication patterns, including games, and works to clarify own communication and validate messages from others. Therapist interprets communication pattern to patient and teaches principles of good communication.

| Behavioral (Bandura, Pavlov, Wolpe, Skinner) | Behavior is learned. Deviation occurs because person has formed undesirable behavioral habits. Because behavior is learned, it can also be unlearned. Deviant behavior may be perpetuated because it reduces anxiety. If so, another anxiety-reducing behavior may be substituted. | Therapy is educational process. Behavioral deviations are not rewarded; more productive behaviors are reinforced. Relaxation therapy and assertiveness training are behavioral approaches. | Patient practices behavioral technique used; does homework and reinforcement exercises. Patient helps develop behavioral hierarchies. Therapist teaches patient about behavioral approach, helps develop behavioral hierarchy, and reinforces desired behaviors. |

Continued

Table 3-1 Models of psychiatric mental health practice—cont'd

Model (Major Theorists)	View of Behavioral Deviation	Therapeutic Process	Roles of Patient and Therapist
Medical (Meyer, Kraeplin, Spitzer, Frances)	Behavioral disruptions result from a biological disease. Symptoms result from a combination of physiological, genetic, environmental, and social factors. Deviant behavior relates to patient's tolerance for stress.	Diagnosis of illness is based on present condition and historical information plus diagnostic studies. Treatment may include somatic and pharmacological therapies in addition to various interpersonal techniques.	Patient practices prescribed therapy regimen and reports effects of therapy to therapist. Patient complies with long-term therapy if necessary. Therapist uses somatic and interpersonal therapies. Therapist diagnoses illness and prescribes therapeutic approach.

(Figure 3-1). The model incorporates the theoretical basis, biopsychosocial components, continuum of coping responses, and nursing activities based on the patient's treatment stage: (1) health promotion, (2) maintenance, (3) acute, or (4) crisis (Figure 3-2). The full model is presented in Figure 3-3 and consists of the following components:

1. *Predisposing factors*—risk factors that influence both the type and the amount of resources the individual can use to cope with stress
2. *Precipitating stressors*—stimuli that the individual perceives as challenging, threatening, or demanding and that require excess energy for coping
3. *Appraisal of stressor*—evaluation of a stressor's significance for the individual's well-being in which the stressor assumes its meaning, intensity, and importance

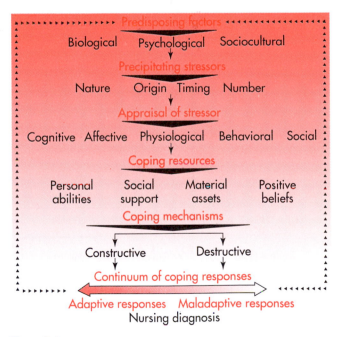

Figure 3-1
Biophysical components of the Stuart Stress Adaptation Model.

TREATMENT STAGE	**CRISIS**
Treatment Goal	Stabilization
Nursing Assessment	Risk Factors
Nursing Intervention	Manage Environment
Expected Outcome	No Harm to Self or Others

TREATMENT STAGE	**ACUTE**
Treatment Goal	Remission
Nursing Assessment	Symptoms and Coping Responses
Nursing Intervention	Mutual Treatment Planning, Modeling, and Teaching
Expected Outcome	Symptom Relief

TREATMENT STAGE	**MAINTENANCE**
Treatment Goal	Recovery
Nursing Assessment	Functional Status
Nursing Intervention	Reinforcement and Advocacy
Expected Outcome	Improved Functioning

TREATMENT STAGE	**HEALTH PROMOTION**
Treatment Goal	Optimal Level of Wellness
Nursing Assessment	Quality of Life and Well-Being
Nursing Intervention	Inspire and Validate
Expected Outcome	Attain Optimal Quality of Life

Figure 3-2
Stages and activities of psychiatric nursing treatment.

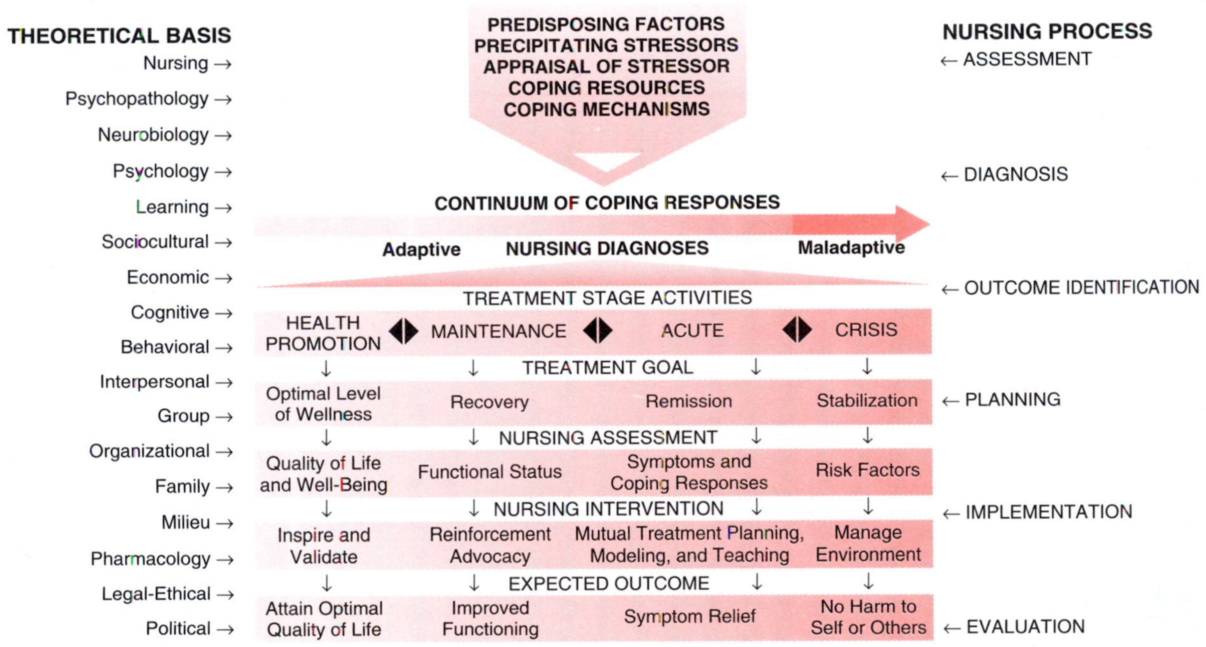

Figure 3-3
The Stuart Stress Adaptation Model of psychiatric nursing care.

4. *Coping resources*—evaluation of the individual's coping options and strategies
5. *Coping mechanisms*—any effort directed at stress management, including direct problem-solving efforts and ego defense mechanisms used to protect the self
6. *Continuum of coping responses*—range of adaptive to maladaptive human responses
7. *Treatment stage activities*—range of nursing functions related to treatment goal, nursing assessment, nursing intervention, and expected outcome

Nursing and Medical Diagnoses

The continuum of coping responses is the subject of nursing diagnoses. The continuum may also include actual health problems that lead to a medical diagnosis. Nursing and medical diagnoses may complement each other, but one is not a component of the other. A patient with one specific medical diagnosis may have a number of complementary nursing diagnoses related to the range of health responses. Conversely, a patient may have a specific nursing diagnosis without any identified medical diagnoses.

Nursing Diagnosis

A nursing diagnosis is a statement of the patient's nursing problem that includes both the adaptive or maladaptive health response and the contributing stressors.

The North American Nursing Diagnosis Association (NANDA) has been identifying, defining, and describing a classification system of nursing diagnoses. Box 3-2 lists the NANDA nursing diagnoses.

Medical Diagnosis

A medical diagnosis is the health problem or disease state of the patient. In the medical model of psychiatry, health problems are the mental disorders classified in the *Diagnostic and Statistical Manual of Mental Disorders,* ed 4 (DSM-IV). In the DSM-IV the individual is evaluated on each of the following axes (Box 3-3):

Axis I   Clinical disorders
Axis II   Personality disorders
Axis III   General medical conditions
Axis IV   Psychosocial and environmental problems
Axis V   Global assessment and functioning

Text continued on p. 66

Box 3-2   NANDA Diagnoses

Activity intolerance
Activity intolerance, risk for
Adaptive capacity: decreased intracranial
Adjustment, impaired
Airway clearance, ineffective
Anxiety
Aspiration, risk for
Body image disturbance
Body temperature, altered, risk for
Bowel incontinence
Breastfeeding, effective
Breastfeeding, ineffective
Breastfeeding, interrupted
Breathing pattern, ineffective
Cardiac output, decreased

Caregiver role strain
Caregiver role strain, risk for
Communication, impaired verbal
Community coping, potential for enhanced
Community coping, ineffective
Confusion, acute
Confusion, chronic
Constipation
Constipation, colonic
Constipation, perceived
Coping, defensive
Coping, family, potential for growth
Coping, ineffective family: compromised

Coping, ineffective family: disabling
Coping, ineffective individual
Decisional conflict (specify)
Denial, ineffective
Diarrhea
Disuse syndrome, risk for
Diversional activity deficit
Dysreflexia
Energy field disturbance
Environmental interpretation syndrome, impaired
Family processes, altered: alcoholism
Family processes, altered

Fatigue
Fear
Fluid volume deficit
Fluid volume deficit, risk for
Fluid volume excess
Gas exchange, impaired
Grieving, anticipatory
Grieving, dysfunctional
Growth and development, altered
Health maintenance, altered
Health-seeking behaviors (specify)
Home maintenance management, impaired
Hopelessness
Hyperthermia
Hypothermia

Continued

Box 3-2   NANDA Diagnoses—cont'd

Incontinence, functional
Incontinence, reflex
Incontinence, stress
Incontinence, total
Incontinence, urge
Infant behavior, disorga-
  nized
Infant behavior, disorga-
  nized: risk for
Infant behavior, orga-
  nized, potential for
  enhanced
Infant feeding pattern,
  ineffective

Management of therapeu-
  tic regimen, individuals:
  ineffective
Memory, impaired
Mobility, impaired
  physical
Noncompliance (specify)
Nutrition, altered: less
  than body requirements
Nutrition, altered: more
  than body requirements
Nutrition, altered risk
  for more than body
  requirements

Rape-trauma syndrome
Rape-trauma syndrome:
  compound reaction
Rape-trauma syndrome:
  silent reaction
Relocation stress syn-
  drome
Role performance, altered
Self-care deficit, bathing/
  hygiene
Self-care deficit, dressing/
  grooming
Self-care deficit, feeding
Self-care deficit, toileting

Spiritual well-being,
  potential for enhanced
Suffocation, risk for
Swallowing, impaired
Thermoregulation, inef-
  fective
Thought processes,
  altered
Tissue integrity, impaired
Tissue perfusion, altered
  (specify): cerebral,
  renal, cardiopulmonary,
  gastrointestinal,
  peripheral

Infection, risk for
Injury, perioperative positioning: risk for
Injury, risk for
Knowledge deficit (specify)
Loneliness, risk for
Management of therapeutic regimen, community: ineffective
Management of therapeutic regimen, families: ineffective
Management of therapeutic regimen, individual: effective

Oral mucous membranes, altered
Pain
Pain, chronic
Parent/infant/child attachment, risk for altered
Parental role conflict
Parenting, altered
Parenting, altered, risk for
Peripheral neurovascular dysfunction, risk for
Personal identity disturbance
Poisoning, risk for
Post-trauma response
Powerlessness
Protection, altered

Self-esteem disturbance
Self-esteem, chronic low
Self-esteem, situational low
Self-mutilation, risk for
Sensory/perceptual alterations (specify)
Sexual dysfunction
Sexuality patterns, altered
Skin integrity, impaired
Skin integrity, impaired, risk for
Sleep pattern disturbance
Social interaction, impaired
Social isolation
Spiritual distress

Trauma, risk for
Unilateral neglect
Urinary elimination, altered
Urinary retention
Ventilation, inability to sustain spontaneous
Ventilatory weaning response, dysfunctional (DVWR)
Violence, risk for: self-directed or directed at others

From North American Nursing Diagnosis Association: NANDA nursing diagnoses: definitions and classification 1997-1998, Philadelphia, 1997, The Association.

Box 3-3   DSM-IV Classification

NOS = Not Otherwise Specified.

An x appearing in a diagnostic code indicates that a specific code number is required.

An ellipsis (. . .) is used in the names of certain disorders to indicate that the name of a specific mental disorder or general medical condition should be inserted when recording the name (e.g., 293.0 Delirium Due to Hypothyroidism).

If criteria are currently met, one of the following severity specifiers may be noted after the diagnosis:
    Mild
    Moderate
    Severe
If criteria are no longer met, one of the following specifiers may be noted:
    In Partial Remission
    In Full Remission
    Prior History

Axis I Clinical Disorders

Disorders usually first diagnosed in infancy, childhood, or adolescence
Mental retardation
Note: These are coded on Axis II.
        317   Mild Mental Retardation
        318.0   Moderate Mental Retardation
        318.1   Severe Mental Retardation
        318.2   Profound Mental Retardation
        319   Mental Retardation, Severity Unspecified
Learning disorders
        315.00 Reading Disorders
        315.1   Mathematics Disorder
        315.2   Disorder of Written Expression
        315.9   Learning Disorder NOS
Motor skills disorder
        315.4   Developmental Coordination Disorder

Box 3-3   DSM-IV Classification—cont'd

Communication disorders

    315.31   Expressive Language Disorder

    315.31   Mixed Receptive-Expressive Language Disorder

    315.39   Phonological Disorder

    307.0   Stuttering

Pervasive developmental disorders

    307.9   Communication Disorder NOS

    299.00   Autistic Disorder

    299.80   Rett's Disorder

    299.10   Childhood Disintegrative Disorder

    299.80   Asperger's Disorder

    299.80   Pervasive Developmental Disorder NOS

Attention-deficit and disruptive behavior disorders

    314.xx   Attention-Deficit/Hyperactivity Disorder

      .01   Combined Type

      .00   Predominantly Inattentive Type

      .01   Predominantly Hyperactive-Impulsive Type

    314.9   Attention-Deficit/Hyperactivity Disorders NOS

    312.8   Conduct Disorder

      Specify type: Childhood-Onset Type/Adolescent-Onset Type

    313.81   Oppositional Defiant Disorder

    312.9   Disruptive Behavior Disorder NOS

Feeding and eating disorders of infancy or early childhood

    307.52   Pica

    307.53   Rumination Disorder

    307.59   Feeding Disorder of Infancy or Early Childhood

Tic disorders

    307.23   Tourette's Disorder

    307.22   Chronic Motor or Vocal Tic Disorder

    307.21   Transient Tic Disorder

      Specify if: Single Episode/Recurrent

    307.20   Tic Disorder NOS

Elimination disorders

    ——.—   Encopresis

    787.6   With Constipation and Overflow Incontinence

Continued

Box 3-3 DSM-IV Classification—cont'd

Elimination disorders—cont'd

307.7   Without Constipation and Overflow Incontinence

307.6   Enuresis (Not Due to a General Medical Condition)
Specify type: Nocturnal Only/Diurnal Only/ Nocturnal and Diurnal

Other disorders of infancy, childhood, or adolescence

309.21 Separation Anxiety Disorder
Specify if: Early Onset

313.89 Reactive Attachment Disorder of Infancy or Early Childhood
Specify type: Inhibited Type/Disinhibited Type

307.3   Stereotypic Movement Disorder
Specify if: With Self-Injurious Behavior

313.9   Disorder of Infancy, Childhood, or Adolescence NOS

Delirium, dementia, amnestic and other cognitive disorders

Delirium

293.0   Delirium Due to . . . [*Indicate the General Medical Condition*]

___._   Substance Intoxication Delirium *(refer to Substance-Related Disorders for substance-specific codes)*

___._   Substance Withdrawal Delirium *(refer to Substance-Related Disorders for substance-specific codes)*

___._   Delirium Due to Multiple Etiologies *(code each of the specific etiologies)*

780.09 Delirium NOS

Dementias

290.xx Dementia of the Alzheimer's Type, With Early Onset *(also code 331.0 Alzheimer's disease on Axis III)*

.10   Uncomplicated

.11   With Delirium

.12   With Delusions

.13   With Depressed Mood
Specify if: With Behavioral Disturbance

Box 3-3   DSM-IV Classification—cont'd

Dementias—cont'd

290.xx   Dementia of the Alzheimer's Type. With Late Onset *(also code 331.0 Alzheimer's disease on Axis III)*
  .0   Uncomplicated
  .3   With Delirium
  .20   With Delusions
  .21   With Depressed Mood
    Specify if: With Behavioral Disturbance

290.xx   Vascular Dementia
  .40   Uncomplicated
  .41   With Delirium
  .42   With Delusions
  .43   With Depressed Mood
    Specify if: With Behavioral Disturbance

294.9   Dementia Due to HIV Disease *(also code 043.1 HIV infection affecting central nervous system on Axis III)*

294.1   Dementia Due to Head Trauma *(also code 854.00 head injury on Axis III)*

294.1   Dementia Due to Parkinson's Disease *(also code 332.0 Parkinson's disease on Axis III)*

294.1   Dementia Due to Huntington's Disease *(also code 333.4 Huntington's disease on Axis III)*

290.10   Dementia Due to Pick's Disease *(also code 331.1 Pick's disease on Axis III)*

290.10   Dementia Due to Creutzfeldt-Jakob Disease *(also code 046.1 Creutzfeldt-Jakob disease on Axis III)*

294.1   Dementia Due to . . . *[indicate the General Medical Condition not listed above] (also code the general medical condition on Axis III)*

——.—   Substance-Induced Persisting Dementia *(refer to Substance-Related Disorders for substance-specific codes)*

——.—   Dementia Due to Multiple Etiologies *(code each of the specific etiologies)*

294.8   Dementia NOS

Continued

Box 3-3   DSM-IV Classification—cont'd

Amnestic disorders

    294.0   Amnestic Disorder Due to . . . *[Indicate the General Medical Condition]*
                Specify if: Transient/Chronic

    ___.__   Substance-Induced Persisting Amnestic Disorder *(refer to Substance-Related Disorders for substance-specific codes)*

    294.8   Amnestic Disorder NOS

Other cognitive disorders

    294.9   Cognitive Disorders NOS

Mental disorders due to a general medical condition not elsewhere classified

    293.89   Catatonic Disorder Due to . . . *[Indicate the General Medical Condition]*

    310.1   Personality Change Due to . . . *[Indicate the General Medical Condition]*
                Specify type: Labile Type/Disinhibited Type/Aggressive Type/Apathetic Type/Paranoid Type/Other Type/Combined Type/Unspecified Type

    293.9   Mental Disorder NOS Due to . . . *[Indicate the General Medical Condition]*

Substance-related disorders

[a]*The following specifiers may be applied to Substance Dependence:*

    With Physiological Dependence/Without Physiological Dependence
    Early Full Remission/Early Partial Remission
    Sustained Full Remission/Sustained Partial Remission
    On Agonist Therapy/In a Controlled Environment

The following specifiers apply to Substance-Induced Disorders as noted:

    [I]With Onset During Intoxication/[W]With Onset During Withdrawal

Alcohol-related disorders

Alcohol use disorders

    303.90   Alcohol Dependence[a]
    305.00   Alcohol Abuse

Alcohol-induced disorders

    303.00   Alcohol Intoxication
    291.8   Alcohol Withdrawal
                Specify if: With Perceptual Disturbances

Box 3-3   DSM-IV Classification—cont'd

Alcohol-induced disorders—cont'd

291.0   Alcohol Intoxication Delirium
291.0   Alcohol Withdrawal Delirium
291.2   Alcohol-Induced Persisting Dementia
291.1   Alcohol-Induced Persisting Amnestic Disorder
291.x   Alcohol-Induced Psychotic Disorder
   .5   With Delusions[I,W]
   .3   With Hallucinations[I,W]
291.8   Alcohol-Induced Mood Disorder[I,W]
291.8   Alcohol-Induced Anxiety Disorder[I,W]
291.8   Alcohol-Induced Sexual Dysfunction[I]
291.8   Alcohol-Induced Sleep Disorder[I,W]
291.9   Alcohol-Related Disorder NOS

Amphetamine (or amphetamine-like)-related disorders

Amphetamine use disorders

304.40   Amphetamine Dependence[a]
305.70   Amphetamine Abuse

Amphetamine-induced disorders

292.89   Amphetamine Intoxication
     Specify if: With Perceptual Disturbances
292.0   Amphetamine Withdrawal
292.81   Amphetamine Intoxication Delirium
292.xx   Amphetamine-Induced Psychotic Disorders
   .11   With Delusions[I]
   .12   With Hallucinations[I]
292.84   Amphetamine-Induced Mood Disorder[I,W]
292.89   Amphetamine-Induced Anxiety Disorder[I]
292.89   Amphetamine-Induced Sexual Dysfunction[I]
292.89   Amphetamine-Induced Sleep Disorder[I,W]
292.9   Amphetamine-Induced Disorder NOS

Caffeine-related disorders

Caffeine-induced disorders

305.90   Caffeine Intoxication
292.89   Caffeine-Induced Anxiety Disorder[I]
292.89   Caffeine-Induced Sleep Disorder[I]
292.9   Caffeine-Related Disorder NOS

Continued

Box 3-3   DSM-IV Classification—cont'd

Cannabis-related disorders
Cannabis use disorders
  304.30 Cannabis Dependence[a]
  305.20 Cannabis Abuse
Cannabis-induced disorders
  292.89 Cannabis Intoxication
     Specify if: Perceptual Disturbances
  292.81 Cannabis Intoxication Delirium
  292.xx Cannabis-Induced Psychotic Disorder
   .11   With Delusions[I]
   .12   With Hallucinations[I]
  292.89 Cannabis-Induced Anxiety Disorder[I]
  292.9   Cannabis-Related Disorder NOS

Cocaine-related disorders
Cocaine use disorders
  304.20 Cocaine Dependence[a]
  305.60 Cocaine Abuse
Cocaine-induced disorders
  292.89 Cocaine intoxication
     Specify if: With Perceptual Disturbances
  292.0   Cocaine Withdrawal
  292.81 Cocaine Intoxication Delirium
  292.xx Cocaine-Induced Psychotic Disorder
   .11   With Delusions[1]
   .12   With Hallucinations[1]
  292.84 Cocaine-Induced Mood Disorder[I,W]
  292.89 Cocaine-Induced Anxiety Disorder[I,W]
  292.89 Cocaine-Induced Sexual Dysfunction[I,W]
  292.89 Cocaine-Induced Sleep Disorder[I,W]
  292.9   Cocaine-Related Disorder NOS

Hallucinogen-related disorders
Hallucinogen use disorders
  304.50 Hallucinogen Dependence[a]
  305.30 Hallucinogen Abuse
Hallucinogen-induced disorders
  292.89 Hallucinogen Intoxication
  292.89 Hallucinogen Persisting Perception Disorder
     (Flashbacks)
  292.81 Hallucinogen Intoxication Delirium

Box 3-3   DSM-IV Classification—cont'd

Hallucinogen-induced disorders—cont'd

    292.xx   Hallucinogen-Induced Psychotic Disorder
            Hallucinogen Intoxication Delirium
       .11   With Delusions[I]
       .12   With Hallucinations[I]
    292.84   Hallucinogen-Induced Mood Disorders[I]
    292.89   Hallucinogen-Induced Anxiety Disorder[I]
    292.9   Hallucinogen-Related Disorder NOS

Inhalant-related disorders

Inhalant use disorders

    304.60   Inhalant Dependence[a]
    305.90   Inhalant Abuse
    292.89   Inhalant Intoxication
    292.81   Inhalant Intoxication Delirium
    292.82   Inhalant-Induced Persisting Dementia
    292.xx   Inhalant-Induced Psychotic Disorder
       .11   With Delusions[I]
       .12   With Hallucinations[I]
    292.84   Inhalant-Induced Mood Disorder
    292.89   Inhalant-Induced Anxiety Disorder
    292.9   Inhalant-Related Disorder NOS

Nicotine-related disorders

Nicotine use disorders

    305.10   Nicotine Dependence[a]

Nicotine-induced disorders

    292.0   Nicotine Withdrawal
    292.9   Nicotine-Related Disorder NOS

Opioid-related disorders

Opioid use disorders

    304.00   Opioid Dependence[a]
    305.50   Opioid Abuse

Opioid-induced disorders

    292.89   Opioid Intoxication
          Specify if: With Perceptual Disturbances
    292.0   Opioid Withdrawal
    292.81   Opioid-Intoxication Delirium
    292.xx   Opioid-Induced Psychotic Disorder
       .11   With Delusions[I]
       .12   With Hallucinations[I]

Continued

Box 3-3   DSM-IV Classification—cont'd

Opioid-induced disorders—cont'd
 292.84 Opioid-Induced Mood Disorder[I]
 292.89 Opioid-Induced Sexual Dysfunction[I,W]
 292.89 Opioid-Induced Sleep Disorder[I]
 292.9 Opioid-Related Disorder NOS
Phencyclidine (or phencyclidine-like)-related disorders
Phencyclidine use disorders
 304.90 Phencyclidine Dependence[a]
 305.90 Phencyclidine Abuse
Phencyclidine-induced disorders
 292.89 Phencyclidine Intoxication
    Specify if: With Perceptual Disturbances
 292.81 Phencyclidine Intoxication Delirium
 292.xx Phencyclidine-Induced Psychotic Disorder
  .11 With Delusions[I]
  .12 With Hallucinations[I]
 292.84 Phencyclidine-Induced Mood Disorder[I]
 292.89 Phencyclidine-Induced Anxiety Disorder[I]
 292.9 Phencyclidine-Related Disorder NOS
Sedative-, hypnotic-, or anxiolytic-related disorders
Sedative, hypnotic, or anxiolytic use disorders
 304.10 Sedative, Hypnotic, or Anxiolytic
    Dependence[a]
 305.40 Sedative, Hypnotic, or Anxiolytic Abuse
Sedative-, hypnotic-, or anxiolytic-induced disorders
 292.89 Sedative, Hypnotic, or Anxiolytic Intoxi-
    cation
 292.0 Sedative, Hypnotic, or Anxiolytic With-
    drawal
    Specify if: With Perceptual Disturbances
 292.81 Sedative, Hypnotic, or Anxiolytic Intoxication
    Delirium
 292.81 Sedative, Hypnotic, or Anxiolytic Withdrawal
    Delirium
 292.82 Sedative-, Hypnotic-, or Anxiolytic-Induced
    Persisting Dementia
 292.83 Sedative-, Hypnotic-, or Anxiolytic-Induced
    Persisting Amnestic Disorder

Box 3-3   DSM-IV Classification—cont'd

Sedative-, hypnotic-, or anxiolytic-induced disorders—cont'd

    292.xx Sedative-, Hypnotic-, or Anxiolytic-Induced Psychotic Disorder

        .11 With Delusions[I,W]
        .12 With Hallucinations[I,W]

    292.84 Sedative-, Hypnotic-, or Anxiolytic-Induced Mood Disorder[I,W]

    292.89 Sedative-, Hypnotic-, or Anxiolytic-Induced Anxiety Disorder[W]

    292.89 Sedative-, Hypnotic-, or Anxiolytic-Induced Sexual Dysfunction[I]

    292.89 Sedative-, Hypnotic-, or Anxiolytic-Induced Sleep Disorder[I,W]

    292.9 Sedative-, Hypnotic-, or Anxiolytic-Related Disorder NOS

Polysubstance-related disorder

    304.80 Polysubstance Dependence[a]

Other (or unknown) substance-related disorders

Other (or unknown) substance use disorders

    304.90 Other (or Unknown) Substance Dependence[a]

    305.90 Other (or Unknown) Substance Abuse

Other (or unknown) substance-induced disorders

    292.89 Other (or Unknown) Substance Intoxication
        Specify if: With Perceptual Disturbances

    292.0 Other (or Unknown) Substance Withdrawal
        Specify if: With Perceptual Disturbances

    292.81 Other (or Unknown) Substance-Induced Delirium

    292.82 Other (or Unknown) Substance-Induced Persisting Dementia

    292.83 Other (or Unknown) Substance-Induced Persisting Amnestic Disorder

    292.xx Other (or Unknown) Substance-Induced Psychotic Disorder

        .11 With Delusions[I,W]
        .12 With Hallucinations[I,W]

Continued

Box 3-3   DSM-IV Classification—cont'd

Other (or unknown) substance-induced disorders—cont'd

292.84   Other (or Unknown) Substance-Induced Mood Disorder[I,W]

292.89   Other (or Unknown) Substance-Induced Anxiety Disorder[I,W]

292.89   Other (or Unknown) Substance-Induced Anxiety Sexual Dysfunction[I]

292.89   Other (or Unknown) Substance-Induced Sleep Disorder[I,W]

292.9   Other (or Unknown) Substance-Related Disorder NOS

Schizophrenia and other psychotic disorders

295.xx   Schizophrenia

The following Classification of Longitudinal Course applies to all subtypes of Schizophrenia:

Episodic With Interepisode Residual Symptoms (*specify if:* With Prominent Negative Symptoms)/ Episodic With No Interepisode Residual Symptoms/ Continuous (*specify if:* With Prominent Negative Symptoms)

Single Episode in Partial Remission (*specify if:* With Prominent Negative Symptoms/Single Episode in Full Remission)

Other or Unspecified Pattern

.30   Paranoid Type

.10   Disorganized Type

.20   Catatonic Type

.90   Undifferentiated Type

.60   Residual Type

295.40   Schizophreniform Disorder
Specify if: Without Good Prognostic Features/With Good Prognostic Features

295.70   Schizoaffective Disorder
Specify type: Bipolar Type/Depressive Type

297.1   Delusional Disorder
Specify type: Erotomanic Type/Grandiose Type/ Jealous Type/Persecutory Type/Somatic Type/ Mixed Type/Unspecified Type

Box 3-3   DSM-IV Classification—cont'd

Schizophrenia and other psychotic disorders—cont'd

298.8   Brief Psychotic Disorder
Specify if: With Marked Stressor(s)/Without Marked Stressor(s)/With Postpartum Onset

297.3   Shared Psychotic Disorder

293.xx   Psychotic Disorder Due to . . . [*Indicate the General Medical Condition*]

.81   With Delusions

.82   With Hallucinations

____.__   Substance-Induced Psychotic Disorder (*refer to Substance-Related Disorders for substance-specific codes*)
Specify if: With Onset During Intoxication/With Onset During Withdrawal

298.9   Psychotic Disorder NOS

Mood disorders

Code current state of Major Depressive Disorder or Bipolar I Disorder in fifth digit:

1 = Mild

2 = Moderate

3 = Severe, Without Psychotic Features

4 = Severe, With Psychotic Features
Specify: Mood-Congruent Psychotic Features/Mood-Incongruent Psychotic Features

5 = In Partial Remission

6 = In Full Remission

0 = Unspecified

The following specifiers apply (for current or most recent episode) to Mood Disorders as noted:

[a]Severity/Psychotic/Remission Specifiers/[b]Chronic/[c]With Catatonic Features/[d]With Melancholic Features/[e]With Atypical Features/[f]With Postpartum Onset

The following specifiers apply to Mood Disorders as noted:

[g]With or Without Full Interepisode Recovery/[h]With Seasonal Pattern/[i]With Rapid Cycling

Depressive disorders

296.xx   Major Depressive Disorder

.2x   Single Episode[a,b,c,d,e,f]

.3x   Recurrent[a,b,c,d,e,f,g,h]

Continued

Box 3-3 DSM-IV Classification—cont'd

Depressive disorders—cont'd

300.4	Dysthymic Disorder	

Specify if: Early Onset/Late Onset
Specify: With Atypical Features

311 Depressive Disorder NOS

Bipolar disorders

296.xx Bipolar I Disorder.
.0x Single Manic Episode[a,c,f]
Specify if: Mixed
.40 Most Recent Episode Hypomanic[g,h,i]
.4x Most Recent Episode Manic[a,c,f,g,h,i]
.6x Most Recent Episode Mixed[a,c,f,g,h,i]
.5x Most Recent Episode Depressed[a,b,c,d,e,f,g,h,i]
.7 Most Recent Episode Unspecified[g,h,i]
296.89 Bipolar II Disorder[a,b,c,d,e,f,g,h,i]
Specify (current or most recent episode):
Hypomanic/Depressed
301.13 Cyclothymic Disorder
296.80 Bipolar Disorder NOS
293.83 Mood Disorder Due to . . . [*Indicate the General Medical Condition*]
Specify type: With Depressive Features/With Major Depressive–Like Episode/With Manic Features/With Mixed Features
——.— Substance-Induced Mood Disorder [*refer to Substance-Related Disorders for substance-specific codes*]
Specify type: With Depressive Features/With Manic Features/With Mixed Features
Specify if: With Onset During Intoxication/With Onset During Withdrawal
296.90 Mood Disorder NOS

Anxiety disorders

300.01 Panic Disorder Without Agoraphobia
300.21 Panic Disorder With Agoraphobia
300.22 Agoraphobia Without History of Panic Disorder
300.29 Specific Phobia
Specify type: Animal Type/Natural Environment Type/Blood-Injection-Injury Type/Situational Type/Other Type

Box 3-3   DSM-IV Classification—cont'd

Anxiety disorders—cont'd

300.23   Social Phobia
Specify if: Generalized

300.3   Obsessive-Compulsive Disorder
Specify if: With Poor Insight

309.81   Posttraumatic Stress Disorder
Specify if: Acute/Chronic
Specify if: With Delayed Onset

308.3   Acute Stress Disorder

300.02   Generalized Anxiety Disorder

293.89   Anxiety Disorder Due to . . . [Indicate the General Medical Condition]
Specify if: With Generalized Anxiety/With Panic Attacks/With Obsessive-Compulsive Symptoms

____.__   Substance-Induced Anxiety Disorder *(refer to Substance-Related Disorders for substance-specific codes)*
Specify if: With Generalized Anxiety/With Panic Attacks/With Obsessive-Compulsive Symptoms/With Phobic Symptoms
Specify if: With Onset During Intoxication/With Onset During Withdrawal

300.00   Anxiety Disorder NOS

Somatoform disorders

300.81   Somatization Disorder

300.81   Undifferentiated Somatoform Disorder

300.11   Conversion Disorder
Specify if: With Motor Symptom or Deficit/With Sensory Symptom or Deficit/With Seizures or Convulsions/With Mixed Presentation

307.xx   Pain Disorder
.80   Associated With Psychological Factors
.89   Associated With Both Psychological Factors and a General Medical Condition
Specify if: Acute/Chronic

300.7   Hypochondriasis
Specify if: With Poor Insight

300.7   Body Dysmorphic Disorder

300.89   Somatoform Disorder NOS

Continued

Box 3-3 DSM-IV Classification—cont'd

Factitious disorders
    300.xx Factitious Disorder
        .16   With Predominantly Psychological Signs and Symptoms
        .19   With Predominantly Physical Signs and Symptoms
        .19   With Combined Psychological and Physical Signs and Symptoms
    300.19 Factitious Disorder NOS

Dissociative disorders
    300.12 Dissociative Amnesia
    300.13 Dissociative Fugue
    300.14 Dissociative Identity Disorder
    300.6   Depersonalization Disorder
    300.15 Dissociative Disorder NOS

Sexual and Gender Identity Disorders
Sexual dysfunctions
The following specifiers apply to all primary Sexual Dysfunctions:
    Lifelong Type/Acquired Type/
    Generalized Type/Situational Type Due to Psychological Factors/Due to Combined Factors

Sexual desire disorders
    302.71 Hypoactive Sexual Desire Disorder
    302.79 Sexual Aversion Disorder

Sexual arousal disorders
    302.72 Female Sexual Arousal Disorder
    302.72 Male Erectile Disorder

Orgasm disorders
    302.73 Female Orgasmic Disorder
    302.74 Male Orgasmic Disorder
    302.75 Premature Ejaculation

Sexual pain disorders
    302.76 Dyspareunia (Not Due to a General Medical Condition)
    306.51 Vaginismus (Not Due to a General Medical Condition)

Sexual dysfunctions due to a general medical condition
    625.8   Female Hypoactive Sexual Desire Disorder Due to . . . [*Indicate the General Medical Condition*]

Box 3-3   DSM-IV Classification—cont'd

Sexual dysfunctions due to a general medical condition—cont'd

609.89 Male Hypoactive Sexual Desire Disorder Due to . . . *[Indicate the General Medical Condition]*

607.84 Male Erectile Disorder Due to . . . *[Indicate the General Medical Condition]*

625.0   Female Dyspareunia Due to . . . *[Indicate the General Medical Condition]*

608.89 Male Dyspareunia Due to . . . *[Indicate the General Medical Condition]*

625.8   Other Female Sexual Dysfunction Due to . . . *[Indicate the General Medical Condition]*

608.89 Other Male Sexual Dysfunction Due to . . . *[Indicate the General Medical Condition]*

___.__   Substance-Induced Sexual Dysfunction (*refer to Substance-Related Disorders for substance-specific codes*)
Specify if: With Impaired Desired/With Impaired Arousal/With Impaired Orgasm/With Sexual Pain
Specify if: With Onset During Intoxication

302.70 Sexual Disfunction NOS

Paraphilias

302.4   Exhibitionism

302.81 Fetishism

302.89 Frotteurism

302.2   Pedophilia
Specify if: Sexually Attracted to Males/Sexually Attracted to Females/Sexually Attracted to Both
Specify type: Exclusive Type/Nonexclusive Type

302.83 Sexual Masochism

302.84 Sexual Sadism

302.3   Transvestic Fetishism
Specify if: With Gender Dysphoria

302.82 Voyeurism

302.9   Paraphilia NOS

Continued

Box 3-3   DSM-IV Classification—cont'd

Gender identity disorder

    3022.xx Gender Identity Disorder

        .6   In Children

        .85   In Adolescents or Adults

           Specify if: Sexually Attracted to Males/Sexually Attracted to Females/Sexually Attracted to Both/Sexually Attracted to Neither

    302.6   Gender Identity Disorder NOS

    302.9   Sexual Disorder NOS

Eating disorders

    307.1   Anorexia nervosa

           Specify type: Restricting Type: Binge-Eating/Purging Type

    307.51 Bulimia Nervosa

           Specify type: Purging Type/Nonpurging Type

    307.50 Eating Disorder NOS

Sleep Disorders

Primary sleep disorders

Dyssomnias

    307.42 Primary Insomnia

    307.44 Primary Hypersomnia

           Specify if: Recurrent

    347   Narcolepsy

    780.59 Breathing-Related Sleep Disorder

    307.45 Circadian Rhythm Sleep Disorder

           Specify type: Delayed Sleep Phase Type/Jet Lag Type/Shift Work Type/Unspecified Type

    307.47 Dyssomnias NOS

Parasomnias

    307.47 Nightmare Disorder

    307.46 Sleep Terror Disorder

    307.46 Sleepwalking Disorder

    307.47 Parasomnia NOS

Sleep disorders related to another mental disorder

    307.42 Insomnia Related to . . . [*Indicate the Axis I or Axis II Disorder*]

    307.44 Hypersomnia Related to . . . [*Indicate the Axis I or Axis II Disorder*]

Box 3-3   DSM-IV Classification—cont'd

Other sleep disorders

780.xx Sleep Disorder Due to . . . [*Indicate the General Medical Condition*]

.52   Insomnia Type

.54   Hypersomnia Type

.59   Parasomnia Type

.59   Mixed Type

___.___   Substance-Induced Sleep Disorder (*refer to Substance-Related Disorders for substance-specific codes*)
Specify type: Insomnia Type/Hypersomnia Type/Parasomnia Type/Mixed Type
Specify if: With Onset During Intoxication/With Onset During Withdrawal

Impulse control disorders not elsewhere classified

312.34 Intermittent Explosive Disorder

312.32 Kleptomania

312.33 Pyromania

312.31 Pathological Gambling

312.39 Trichotillomania

312.30 Impulse Control Disorder NOS

Adjustment disorders

309.xx Adjustment Disorder

.0   With Depressed Mood

.24   With Anxiety

.28   With Mixed Anxiety and Depressed Mood

.3   With Disturbance of Conduct

.4   With Mixed Disturbance of Emotions and Conduct

.9   Unspecified
Specify if: Acute/Chronic

Personality disorders

Note: These are coded on Axis II.

301.0   Paranoid Personality Disorder

301.20 Schizoid Personality Disorder

301.22 Schizotypal Personality Disorder

301.7   Antisocial Personality Disorder

301.83 Borderline Personality Disorder

301.50 Histrionic Personality Disorder

Continued

Box 3-3   DSM-IV Classification—cont'd

Personality disorders—cont'd

    301.81 Narcissistic Personality Disorder
    301.82 Avoidant Personality Disorder
    301.6   Dependent Personality Disorder
    301.4   Obsessive-Compulsive Personality Disorder
    301.9   Personality Disorder NOS

Other conditions that may be a focus of clinical attention

Psychological factors affecting medical condition

    316   ... [*Specified Psychological Factor*] ...
            affecting [*Indicate the General Medical
            Condition*] *Choose name based on nature
            of factors:*
            Mental Disorder Affecting Medical Condition
            Psychological Symptoms Affecting Medical
            Condition
            Personality Traits or Coping Style Affecting
            Medical Condition
            Maladaptive Health Behaviors Affecting
            Medical Condition
            Stress-Related Physiological Response
            Affecting Medical Condition
            Other or Unspecified Psychological Factors
            Affecting Medical Condition

Medication-induced movement disorders

    332.1   Neuroleptic-Induced Parkinsonism
    333.92 Neuroleptic Malignant Syndrome
    333.7   Neuroleptic-Induced Acute Dystonia
    333.99 Neuroleptic-Induced Acute Akathisia
    333.82 Neuroleptic-Induced Tardive Dyskinesia
    333.1   Medication-Induced Postural Tremor
    333.90 Medication-Induced Movement Disorder NOS

Other medication-induced disorders

    995.2   Adverse Effects of Medication NOS

Relational problems

    V61.9   Relational Problem Related to a Mental
            Disorder or General Medical Condition
    V61.20 Parent-Child Relational Problem
    V61.1   Partner Relational Problem
    V61.8   Sibling Relational Problem
    V62.81 Relational Problem NOS

Box 3-3   DSM-IV Classification—cont'd

Problems related to abuse or neglect

V61.21 Physical Abuse of Child (*code 995.5 if focus of attention is on victim*)

V61.21 Sexual Abuse of Child (*code 995.5 if focus of attention is on victim*)

V61.21 Neglect of Child (*code 995.5 if focus of attention is on victim*)

V61.1 Physical Abuse of Adult (*code 995.81 if focus of attention is on victim*)

V61.1 Sexual Abuse of Adult (*code 995.81 if focus of attention is on victim*)

Additional conditions that may be a focus of clinical attention

V15.81 Noncompliance With Treatment
V65.2 Malingering
V71.01 Adult Antisocial Behavior
V71.02 Childhood or Adolescent Antisocial Behavior
V62.89 Borderline Intellectual Functioning
Note: This is coded on Axis II.
780.9 Age-Related Cognitive Decline
V62.82 Bereavement
V62.3 Academic Problem
V62.2 Occupational Problem
313.82 Identity Problem
V62.89 Religious or Spiritual Problem
V62.4 Acculturation Problem
V62.89 Phase of Life Problem

Additional codes

300.9 Unspecified Mental Disorder (nonpsychotic)
V71.09 No Diagnosis or Condition on Axis I
799.9 Diagnosis or Condition Deferred on Axis I
V71.09 No Diagnosis on Axis II
799.9 Diagnosis Deferred on Axis II

Axis II Personality Disorders

301.0 Paranoid Personality Disorder
301.20 Schizoid Personality Disorder

Continued

Box 3-3 DSM-IV Classification—cont'd

Axis II Personality Disorders—cont'd

301.22 Schizotypal Personality Disorder
301.7   Antisocial Personality Disorder
301.83 Borderline Personality Disorder
301.5   Histrionic Personality Disorder
301.81 Narcissistic Personality Disorder
301.82 Avoidant Personality Disorder
301.65 Dependent Personality Disorder
301.45 Obsessive-Compulsive Personality Disorder
301.9   Personality Disorder NOS

Axis III General Medical Conditions (with ICD-9-CM codes)

Infectious and Parasitic Diseases (001-139)
Neoplasms (140-239)
Endocrine, Nutritional, and Metabolic Diseases and Immunity Disorders (240-279)
Diseases of the Blood and Blood-Forming Organs (280-289)
Diseases of the Nervous System and Sense Organs (320-389)
Diseases of the Circulatory System (390-459)
Diseases of the Respiratory System (460-519)
Diseases of the Digestive System (520-579)
Diseases of the Genitourinary System (580-629)
Complications of Pregnancy, Childbirth, and the Puerperium (630-676)
Diseases of the Skin and Subcutaneous Tissue (680-709)
Diseases of the Musculoskeletal System and Connective Tissue (710-739)
Congenital Anomalies (740-759)
Certain Conditions Originating in the Perinatal Period (760-779)
Symptoms, Signs, and Ill-Defined Conditions (780-799)
Injury and Poisoning (800-999)

Box 3-3   DSM-IV Classification—cont'd

Axis IV Psychosocial and Environmental Problems

- **Problems with primary support group**—e.g., death of a family member; health problems in family; disruption of family by separation, divorce, or estrangement; removal from the home; remarriage of parent; sexual or physical abuse; parental overprotection; neglect of child; inadequate discipline; discord with siblings; birth of a sibling
- **Problems related to the social environment**—e.g., death or loss of friend; inadequate social support; living alone; difficulty with acculturation; discrimination; adjustment to life cycle transition (e.g., retirement)
- **Educational problems**—e.g., illiteracy; academic problems; discord with teachers or classmates; inadequate school environment
- **Occupational problems**—e.g., unemployment; threat of job loss; stressful work schedule; difficult work conditions; job dissatisfaction; job change; discord with boss or co-workers
- **Housing problems**—e.g., homelessness; inadequate housing; unsafe neighborhood; discord with neighbors or landlord
- **Economic problems**—e.g., extreme poverty; inadequate finances; insufficient welfare support
- **Problems with access to health care services**—e.g., inadequate health care services; transportation to health care facilities unavailable; inadequate health insurance
- **Problems related to interaction with the legal system crime**—e.g., arrest; incarceration; litigation; victim of crime

Continued

Box 3-3 DSM-IV Classification—cont'd

Axis V Global Assessment of Functioning (GAF) Scale[*]

Consider psychological, social, and occupational functioning on a hypothetical continuum of mental health-illness. Do not include impairment in functioning due to physical (or environmental) limitations.

Code (*Note:* Use intermediate codes when appropriate, e.g., 45, 68, 72.)

100 | Superior functioning in a wide range of activities, life's problems never seem to get out of hand, is sought out by others because of many positive
91 | qualities. No symptoms.

90 | Absent or minimal symptoms (e.g., mild anxiety before an exam), good functioning in all areas, interested and involved in a wide range of activities, socially effective, generally satisfied with life, no more than everyday problems or concerns (e.g., an occasional argument with family
81 | members).

80 | If symptoms are present, they are transient and expectable reactions to psychosocial stressors (e.g., difficulty concentrating after family argument); no more than slight impairment in social, occupational, or school functioning (e.g., temporarily falling
71 | behind in schoolwork).

[*]The rating of overall psychological functioning on a scale of 0-100 was operationalized by Luborsky in the Health-Sickness Rating Scale (Luborsky L: Clinicians' judgments of mental health, *Arch Gen Psychiatry* 7:407-417, 1962). Spitzer and colleagues developed a revision of the Health-Sickness Rating Scale called the Global Assessment Scale (GAS) (Endicott J, Spitzer RL, Fleiss JL, Cohen J: The global assessment scale, a procedure for measuring overall severity of psychiatric disturbance, *Arch Gen Psychiatry* 33:766-771, 1976). A modified version of the GAS was included in DSM-III-R as the Global Assessment of Functioning (GAF) Scale.

Box 3-3   DSM-IV Classification—cont'd

Code

70   Some mild symptoms (e.g., depressed mood and mild insomnia) OR some difficulty in social, occupational, or school functioning (e.g., occasional truancy, theft within the household), but generally functioning pretty well, has some meaningful
61   interpersonal relationships.

60   Moderate symptoms (e.g., flat affect and circumstantial speech, occasional panic attacks) OR moderate difficulty in social, occupational, or school functioning (e.g., few friends, conflicts
51   with peers or co-workers).

50   Serious symptoms (e.g., suicidal ideation, severe obsessional rituals, frequent shoplifting) OR any serious impairment in social, occupational, or school functioning (e.g., no friends, unable to
41   keep a job).

40   Some impairment in reality testing or communication (e.g., speech is at times illogical, obscure, or irrelevant) OR major impairment in several areas, such as work or school, family relations, judgment, thinking, or mood (e.g., depressed man avoids friends, neglects family, and is unable to work; child frequently beats up younger children, is defiant at home, and is failing at school).
31

30   Behavior is considerably influenced by delusions or hallucinations OR serious impairment in communication or judgment (e.g., sometimes incoherent, acts grossly inappropriately, suicidal preoccupation) OR inability to function in almost all areas (e.g.,
21   stays in bed all day; no job, home, or friends).

Continued

Box 3-3   DSM-IV Classification—cont'd

Code

20   Some danger of hurting self or others (e.g., suicide attempts without clear expectation of death, frequently violent, manic excitement) OR occasionally fails to maintain minimal personal hygiene (e.g., smears feces) OR gross impairment in
11   communication (e.g., largely incoherent or mute).

10   Persistent danger of severely hurting self or others (e.g., recurrent violence) OR persistent inability to maintain minimal personal hygiene OR serious
1   suicidal act with clear expectation of death.

0   Inadequate information.

From American Psychiatric Association: *Diagnostic and statistical manual of mental disorders,* ed 4 (DSM-IV), Washington, DC, 1994, The Association.

your **INTERNET**
c o n n e c t i o n

Mental Health Net: http://www.cmhcsys.com
PsychLink: http://www.psychlink.com

Suggested readings

Albert G: What are the characteristics of effective psychotherapists? The experts speak, *J Pract Psych Behav Health* 3:36, 1997.

Alexander J et al: Determinants of mental health providers' expectations of patients' improvement, *Psychiatric Serv* 48:671, 1997.

Blair T: The placebogenic phenomenon: Art in psychiatic nursing, *J Psychosoc Nurs* 34:11, 1996.

Cohen C: The political and moral economy of mental health, *Psychiatric Serv* 48:768, 1997.

Frances A, First M, Pincus H: DSM-IV: its value and limitations, *Harvard Mental Health Letter,* 4, June 1995.

Gabbard G et al: The economic impact of psychotherapy: a review, *Am J Psychiatry 154:147, 1997.*

Gross D, Fogg L, Conrad B: Designing interventions in psychosocial research, *Arch Psychiatric Nurs* 7:259, 1993.

Hollingsworth E, Sweeney J: Mental health expenditures for services for people with severe mental illness, *Psychiatric Serv* 48:485, 1997.

Hoyt M: *Brief therapy and managed care: readings for contemporary practice,* San Francisco, 1995, Jossey-Bass.

Kessler C, Gordon L: *Measuring stress: a guide for health and social scientists,* New York, 1995, Oxford University Press.

Stuart G, Laraia M: *Principles and practice of psychiatric nursing,* ed 6, St Louis, 1998, Mosby.

Stuhlmiller C: The construction of disorders, *J Psychosoc Nurs* 33:20, 1995.

Thompson J: Trends in the development of psychiatric services, 1844–1994, *Hosp Comm Psychiatry* 45:987, 1994.

Wahl O: *Media madness: public images of mental illness,* New Brunswick, New Jersey, 1995, Rutgers University Press.

Biopsychosocial Context of Psychiatric Nursing Care

4

The practice of contemporary psychiatric nursing requires that the nurse use a model of care that integrates the biological, psychological, and sociocultural aspects of the individual in assessing, planning, and implementing nursing interventions.

Biological Context of Care

New tools and techniques help to explain how the brain works and the brain, mind, and body interact. The psychiatric nurse must have a working knowledge of the normal structure and function of the brain, particularly mental functions, just as the cardiac care nurse must know how the heart works. Psychiatric nurses can then interpret expanding biological information and its potential for effective treatments to consumers of mental health services and to other health-care providers, thus further reinforcing nurses' role as patient advocates.

Neuroimaging Techniques

Brain imaging techniques allow for direct viewing of the structure and function of the intact, living brain. These techniques not only help in diagnosing some brain disorders but also map the regions of the brain and correlate them with function. They provide pictures of the working brain. Table 4-1 describes some of these important imaging techniques.

Table 4-1   Brain imaging techniques

Technique	How it Works	What it Images
Computed tomography (CT)	Series of x-rays are computer-constructed into "slices" of the brain that can be stacked by the computer, giving a three-dimensional view.	Brain structure
Magnetic resonance imaging (MRI)	Magnetic field surrounding the head induces brain tissues to emit radio waves that are computerized for clear, detailed construction of sectional images of the brain.	Brain structure; newer functional MRI (FMRI) techniques show brain activity
Brain electrical activity mapping (BEAM)	CT techniques are used to display data derived from electro-encephalographic (EEG) recordings of brain electrical activity that can be sensory-evoked by specific stimuli (e.g., flash of light, sudden sound) or cognitive-evoked by specific mental tasks.	Brain activity/function
Positron emission tomography (PET)	Injected radioactive substance travels to the brain and shows up as a bright spot on the scan; different substances are taken up by the brain in different amounts, depending on type of tissue and level of activity.	Brain activity/function
Single-photon emission computed tomography (SPECT)	Similar to PET, but SPECT uses more stable substances and different detectors to visualize blood flow patterns.	Brain activity/function

Genetics of Mental Illness

The ongoing search for the gene or genes that cause mental illness has been difficult. The only gene that has been linked to any mental illness causes the development of Alzheimer's disease in about 10% of people with the disorder.

Current information regarding the transmission of mental illness is primarily based on investigations into human inheritance. The three types of studies in this area follow:

1. *Adoption studies,* which compare a trait among biological versus adoptive family members or other control groups
2. *Twin studies,* which compare how often identical twins, who are genetically identical, and fraternal twins, who have the genetic similarity of nontwin siblings, are concordant for a trait
3. *Family studies,* which compare whether a trait is more common among first-degree relatives, such as parents, siblings, and other offspring, than it is among more distant relatives or control groups

Circadian Rhythms

Recent biological research has suggested that body rhythms are governed by internal circadian pacemakers located in specific areas of the brain and that they are subject to change by specific external cues. Circadian rhythm is like a network of internal clocks that time and coordinate events within the body according to an approximate 24-hour cycle. These rhythms affect every aspect of health and well-being, including lifestyle, sleep, moods, eating, drinking, fertility, and illness. Recent research suggests that one of the most important internal timekeepers is located in the hypothalamus of the brain.

Psychoimmunology

Psychoimmunology is a relatively new field that explores the psychological influences on the nervous system's control of immune responsiveness. Although the evidence is compelling that psychosocial stressors can temporarily impair the immune response and thus contribute to the development of a variety of illnesses, the role for autoimmunity in the major psychiatric illnesses is unclear. Efforts to relate specific stressors to specific diseases have not generally been successful, but stress is recognized as a potential key to understanding the development and course of many illnesses.

Biological Assessment of the Psychiatric Patient

Psychiatric nurses should include a thorough biological assessment in their evaluation of psychiatric patients. Undiagnosed physical illness can be costly and dangerous if undetected or treated incorrectly. The psychiatric nurse is well suited to screen for the major signs of physical or organic disorders that may complicate a patient's psychiatric status, to identify physical illnesses that may have been overlooked, or to refer a patient for a thorough medical diagnostic work-up if indicated.

A complete health-care history of the patient, lifestyle review, physical examination, analysis of laboratory values, and discussion of presenting symptoms and coping responses are essential elements of a baseline assessment (Box 4-1). The nurse should be able to perform a basic physical examination to assess for gross abnormalities and be able to interpret the results of existing, more complex examinations. Appearance, gait, coordination, bilateral strength, tremors and tics, speech, and symptoms such as headaches, blurred vision, dizziness, vomiting, motor weakness, disorientation, confusion, and memory problems should be assessed in detail.

Only after a patient has been carefully screened can the nurse determine which of the patient's presenting problems are amenable to psychiatric intervention and which may require a consultant in another specialty.

Psychological Context of Care

All nurses, regardless of clinical setting, should be proficient in assessing a patient's psychological status and should incorporate the findings in the patient's plan of care. The mental status examination is a cornerstone in the evaluation of any patient with a medical, neurological, or psychiatric disorder that affects thoughts, emotions, or behavior. It is used to detect changes or abnormalities in a person's intellectual functioning, thought content, judgment, mood, and affect and can be used to suggest possible brain lesions. In this way the mental status exam is to

Box 4-1   Biological Assessment of the Psychiatric Patient

Health Care History

General health care

Regular and specialty health-care providers

Frequency of health-care visits

Last medical examination and test results

Any unusual circumstances of birth, including mother's preterm habits and condition

Hospitalizations and surgeries

When; why indicated; treatments; outcome

Brain impairment

Diagnosed brain problem

Head trauma

Details of accidents or periods of unconsciousness for any reason: blows to head, electrical shocks, high fevers, seizures, fainting, dizziness, headaches, falls

Cancer

Full history, particularly metastases (lung, breast, melanoma, gastrointestinal tract, and kidney are most likely to metastasize)

Results of treatment (chemotherapy, surgeries)

Lung problems

Details of any condition or event that restricts airflow to lungs for more than 2 minutes or adversely affects oxygen absorption (brain uses 20% of oxygen in body), such as with chronic obstructive pulmonary disease, near drowning, near strangulation, high-altitude oxygen deprivation, resuscitation events

Cardiac problems

Childhood illnesses such as scarlet or rheumatic fever

History of heart attacks, strokes, or hypertension

Blood diseases

Anemia resulting in hypoxia

Arteriosclerotic conditions

Human immunodeficiency virus (HIV)

Diabetes

Stability of glucose levels

Endocrine disturbances

Thyroid and adrenal function particularly

Reproductive history
Menstrual history

Lifestyle

Eating
Details of unusual or unsupervised diets, appetite, weight changes, cravings, and caffeine intake

Medications
Full history of current and past psychiatric medications given to patient and first-degree relatives

Substance use
Alcohol and drug use

Toxins
Overcome by automobile exhaust or natural gas
Exposure to lead, mercury, insecticides, herbicides, solvents, cleaning agents, lawn chemicals

Occupation (current and past)
Chemicals in workplace (e.g., farming, painting)
Work-related accidents (e.g., construction, mining)
Military experiences
Stressful job circumstances

Injury
Safe sex practices
Contact sports and sports-related injuries
Exposure to violence or abuse

Impact of culture
Age, ethnicity, gender, education, income, belief system

Physical Examination

Current health statistics
Immunizations
Allergies
Last physical examination and Pap smear

Review of physiological systems
Integumentary: skin, nails, hair, scalp
Head: eyes, ears, nose, mouth, throat, neck
Breasts
Respiratory
Cardiovascular
Hematolymphatic
Gastrointestinal tract

Continued

Box 4-1   Biological Assessment of the Psychiatric Patient—cont'd

Physical Examination—cont'd

Urinary tract
Genital
Neurological
Musculoskeletal
Nutritive
Restorative: sleep and rest
Endocrine
Allergic and immunological

Laboratory Values

Blood, plasma, serum
Urine
Steroid hormones
Polypeptide hormones
Thyroid hormones
Hematology
Cerebrospinal fluid

Presenting Symptoms and Coping Responses

Description: nature, frequency, intensity
Threats to safety of self or others
Functional status
Quality of life

psychiatric nursing what the physical exam is to general medical nursing.

Interviewing Skills

The goal-directed patient interview can be facilitated in the following ways:

1. Address the patient by name and introduce yourself and the purpose of the interview.
2. Demonstrate awareness of and respect for the patient and a sensitivity to the patient's feelings by assuming a warm, empathic approach.
3. Select an environment that provides privacy, physical comfort, and minimum distractions.
4. Listen to what the patient is saying as well as to underlying themes and omissions.
5. Observe verbal content and nonverbal communication.
6. Allow sufficient time for the interview and avoid a tense, hurried approach.
7. Monitor your feelings and anxieties in the patient interview.
8. Use secondary sources of information (e.g., medical history, psychological evaluation, social history) as a supplement to, not a substitute for, your clinical impressions and evaluation.

Mental Status Examination

The mental status exam represents a cross section of the patient's psychological life and the sum of the nurse's observations and impressions at that moment. It is not an evaluation of how that patient was in the past or will be in the future. The examination is an evaluation of the patient's current state. The elements of the exam depend on the patient's clinical presentation, as well as the patient's educational and cultural background. It includes observing the patient's behavior and describing it in an objective, nonjudgmental manner. The mental status exam includes information pertaining to the categories listed in Box 4-2.

Appearance

In the mental status examination the nurse notes the patient's general appearance.

Box 4-2   Categories of the Mental Status Examination

General Description

Appearance
Speech
Motor activity
Interaction during interview

Emotional State

Mood
Affect

Experiences

Perceptions

Thinking

Thought content
Thought process

Sensorium and Cognition

Level of consciousness
Memory
Level of concentration and calculation
Information and intelligence
Judgment
Insight

Observations

Areas that should be included are the following physical characteristics of the patient:

- Apparent age
- Manner of dress
- Cleanliness
- Posture
- Unusual gait
- Facial expressions
- Eye contact
- Pupil dilation or constriction
- General state of health and nutrition

NURSE ALERT. Dilated pupils are sometimes associated with drug intoxication, whereas pupil constriction may indicate narcotic addiction. Stooped posture is often seen in depressed individuals. Manic patients may dress in colorful or unusual attire.

Speech

Speech is usually described in terms of rate, volume, and characteristics. *Rate* refers to the speed of the patient's speech, and *volume* refers to how loudly a patient talks.

Observations

Speech can be described as follows:

- Rate—rapid or slow
- Volume—loud or soft
- Amount—minimal (paucity), mute, or pressured
- Characteristics—stuttering, slurring of words, or unusual accents

NURSE ALERT. Speech disturbances are often caused by specific brain disturbances. For example, mumbling may occur in patients with Huntington's chorea, and slurring of speech in intoxicated patients. Manic patients often show pressured speech, and depressed patients often have paucity of speech.

Motor activity

Motor activity is concerned with the patient's physical movement.

Observations

The nurse should record the following:

- Level of activity—lethargic, tense, restless, or agitated
- Type of activity—tics, grimaces, or tremors
- Unusual gestures or mannerisms—compulsions

NURSE ALERT. Excessive body movement may be associated with anxiety, mania, or stimulant abuse. Minimal
body activity may suggest depression, organicity, catatonic schizophrenia, or drug-induced stupor. Tics and grimaces may suggest adverse effects to medications. Repeated
motor movements or compulsions may indicate obsessive-
compulsive disorder. Repeated picking of lint or dirt off
clothing is sometimes associated with delirium or toxic
conditions.

Interaction during the interview

Interaction describes how the patient relates to the nurse during the
interview.

Observations

Has the patient been hostile, uncooperative, irritable, guarded,
apathetic, defensive, suspicious, or seductive? The nurse may
explore this area by asking: "You seem irritated about something;
is that an accurate observation?"

NURSE ALERT. Suspiciousness may be evident in the paranoid or substance-abusing patient. Irritability may suggest an
anxiety disorder. Apathy may be associated with depression,
and seductive behavior with bipolar illness.

Mood

Mood is the patient's self-report of the prevailing emotional state
and reflects the patient's life situation.

Observations

Mood can be evaluated by asking a simple, nonleading question
such as, "How are you feeling today?" Does the patient report
feeling sad, fearful, hopeless, euphoric, or anxious? Asking the
patient to rate mood on a scale of 0 to 10 can help provide the nurse
with an immediate reading of the patient's mood.

If the potential for suicide is suspected, it is essential that the nurse inquire directly regarding the patient's thoughts about self-destruction. Suicidal and homicidal thoughts must be addressed directly. To judge a patient's suicidal or homicidal risk, the nurse should assess the patient's plans, ability to carry out those plans (e.g., availability of guns), the patient's attitude about death, and available support systems.

NURSE ALERT. Most people with depression describe feeling hopeless, and 25% of those with depression have suicidal ideation. Suicidal ideation is also common in patients with anxiety disorders and schizophrenia. Elation is most common in those with mania.

Affect

Affect is the patient's prevailing emotional tone observed by the nurse during the interview.

Observations
Affect can be described in terms of the following:
- Range
- Duration
- Intensity
- Appropriateness

Does the patient report significant life events without any emotional response, indicating flat affect? Does the patient's response appear restricted or blunted in some way? Does the patient demonstrate great lability in expression by shifting from one affect to another quickly? Is the patient's response incongruent with speech content? For example, does the patient report being persecuted by the police and then laugh?

NURSE ALERT. Labile affect is often seen in manic patients, and a flat, incongruent affect is often evident in schizophrenic patients.

Perceptions

The two major types of perceptual problems are hallucinations and illusions. *Hallucinations* are defined as false sensory impressions or experiences. *Illusions* are false perceptions or false responses to a sensory stimulus.

Observations

Hallucinations may occur in any of the five major sensory modalities, as follows:

- Auditory (sound)
- Visual (sight)
- Tactile (touch)
- Gustatory (taste)
- Olfactory (smell)

Command hallucinations are those that tell the person to do something, such as kill oneself, harm another, or join someone in the afterlife. The nurse might inquire about the patient's perceptions by asking, "Do you ever see or hear things?" or "Do you have strange experiences as you fall asleep or on awakening?"

> **NURSE ALERT.**   Auditory hallucinations are the most common and suggest schizophrenia. Visual hallucinations suggest organicity. Tactile hallucinations suggest organic mental disorder, cocaine abuse, and delirium tremens.

Thought content

Thought content refers to the specific meaning expressed in the patient's communication, or the "what" of the patient's thinking.

Observations

Although the patient may talk about a variety of subjects during the interview, the nurse should note several content areas in the mental status examination (Box 4-3). They may be complicated and are often concealed by the patient.

Box 4-3 Thought Content Descriptors

Delusion—false belief that is firmly maintained even though it is not shared by others and is contradicted by social reality

Religious delusion—belief that one is favored by a higher being or is an instrument of that being

Somatic delusion—belief that one's body or parts of one's body are diseased or distorted

Grandiose delusion—belief that one possesses greatness or special powers

Paranoid delusion—excessive or irrational suspiciousness and distrustfulness of others, characterized by systematized delusions that others are "out to get them" or are spying on them

Thought broadcasting—delusion about thoughts being aired to the outside world

Thought insertion—delusion that thoughts are placed into the mind by outside people or influences

Depersonalization—feeling of having lost self-identity and that things around the person are different, strange, or unreal

Hypochondriasis—somatic overconcern with and morbid attention to details of body functioning

Ideas of reference—incorrect interpretation of casual incidents and external events as having direct personal references

Magical thinking—belief that thinking equates with doing; characterized by lack of realistic relationship between cause and effect

Nihilistic ideas—thoughts of nonexistence and hopelessness

Obsession—idea, emotion, or impulse that repetitively and insistently forces itself into consciousness, although it is unwelcome

Phobia—morbid fear associated with extreme anxiety

NURSE ALERT. Obsessions and phobias are symptoms associated with anxiety disorders. Delusions, depersonalization, and ideas of reference suggest schizophrenia and other psychotic disorders.

Thought process

Thought process refers to the "how" of the patient's self-expression. A patient's thought process is observed through speech. The patterns or forms of verbalization rather than the content are assessed.

Observations

A number of problems can be assessed that involve a patient's thinking (Box 4-4). The nurse can ask various questions to evaluate the patient's thought process. Does the patient's thinking proceed in a systematic, organized, and logical manner? Is the patient's self-expression clear? Is it relatively easy for the patient to move from one topic to another?

NURSE ALERT. Circumstantial thinking may be a sign of defensiveness or paranoid thinking. Loose associations and neologisms suggest schizophrenia or other psychotic disorders. Flight of ideas indicates mania. Perseveration is often associated with brain damage and psychotic disorders. Word salad represents the highest level of thought disorganization. (See Box 4-4.)

Level of consciousness

Mental status examinations routinely assess a patient's orientation to the current situation.

Observations

A variety of terms can be used to describe a patient's level of consciousness, such as confused, sedated, or stuporous. In addition, the patient should be questioned regarding orientation to time,

Box 4-4   Thought Process Descriptors

Circumstantial—thought and speech associated with excessive and unnecessary detail that is usually relevant to a question, and an answer is ultimately given

Flight of ideas—overproductive speech characterized by rapid shifting from one topic to another and fragmented ideas

Loose associations—lack of a logical relationship between thoughts and ideas that renders speech and thought inexact, vague, diffuse, and unfocused

Neologisms—new word or words created by patient, which are often a blend of other words

Perseveration—involuntary, excessive continuation or repetition of a single response, idea, or activity; may apply to speech or movement, but most often verbal

Tangential—similar to circumstantial, but patient never returns to central point and never answers original question

Thought blocking—sudden stopping in the train of thought or in midst of a sentence

Word salad—series of words that seem completely unrelated

place, and person. The nurse usually can determine this by the patient's answers to the following three simple questions:

1. *Person*—What is your name?
2. *Place*—Where are you today (e.g., what city, what particular building)?
3. *Time*—What is today's date?

If the patient answers correctly, the nurse can note "oriented times three." Level of orientation can also be pursued in greater depth, but this area may be confounded by sociocultural factors.

NURSE ALERT.   Patients with organic mental disorder may give grossly inaccurate answers, with orientation to person remaining intact longer than orientation to time or place. Patients with schizophrenic disorders may say they are someone else or somewhere else or reveal a personalized orientation to the world.

Memory

A mental status examination can provide a quick screen of potential memory problems but not a definitive answer to whether a specific impairment exists. Neuropsychological assessment is required to specify the nature and extent of memory impairment. Memory is broadly defined as the ability to recall past experiences.

Observations

The following areas must be tested:
- *Remote memory*—recall of events, information, and people from the distant past
- *Recent memory*—recall of events, information, and people from the past week or so
- *Immediate memory*—recall of information or data to which a person was just exposed

Recall of remote events involves reviewing information from the patient's history. This part of the evaluation can be woven into the history-taking portion of the nursing assessment. This involves asking the patient questions about time and place of birth, names of schools attended, date of marriage, ages of family members, and so forth. The problem with an evaluation of the patient's remote memory is that the nurse is often unable to tell if the patient is reporting events accurately. Thus the nurse may need to check past records or have family or friends confirm this historical information.

Recent memory can be tested by asking the patient to recall the events of the past 24 hours. A reliable informant may be needed to verify this information. Another test of recent memory is to ask the patient to remember three words (e.g., object, color, address) and then repeat them 15 minutes later in the interview.

Immediate recall can be tested by asking the patient to repeat a series of numbers either forward or backward within 10 seconds. The nurse should begin with a short series of numbers and proceed to longer lists.

> **NURSE ALERT.** Loss of memory occurs with organicity, dissociative disorder, and conversion disorder. Alzheimer's dementia patients retain remote memory longer than recent memory. Anxiety and depression can impair immediate retention and recent memory.

Level of concentration and calculation

Concentration is the patient's ability to pay attention during the course of the interview. Calculation is the person's ability to do simple math.

Observations

The nurse should note the patient's level of distractibility. Calculation can be assessed by asking the patient to do the following:

1. Count from 1 to 20 rapidly.
2. Do simple calculations, such as 2×3 or $21 + 7$.
3. Serially subtract 7 from 100.

If patients have difficulty subtracting 7 from 100, they can be asked to subtract 3 from 20 in the same way. Finally, more functional calculation skills can be assessed by asking practical questions such as, "How many nickels are there in $1.35?"

> **NURSE ALERT.** Many psychiatric illnesses impair the ability to concentrate and complete simple calculations. It is particularly important to differentiate among organic mental disorder, anxiety, and depression.

Information and intelligence

Information and intelligence are controversial areas of assessment, and the nurse should be cautious about judging intelligence after a brief and limited contact typical of the mental status examination. The nurse should also remember that information in this category is highly influenced by sociocultural factors of the nurse, the patient, and the treatment setting.

Observations

The nurse should assess the last grade of school completed, the patient's general fund of knowledge, and use of vocabulary. It is also critical that the nurse assess the patient's level of literacy. The ability to conceptualize and abstract can be tested by having the patient explain a series of proverbs. The patient can be given an example of a proverb with its interpretation and then asked to explain what several proverbs mean. Frequently used proverbs include the following:

- When it rains, it pours.
- A stitch in time saves nine.
- A rolling stone gathers no moss.
- The proof of the pudding is in the eating.
- People who live in glass houses shouldn't throw stones.
- A bird in the hand is worth two in the bush.

If the patient's educational level is below the eighth grade, asking the patient to list similarities between a series of paired objects may better help the nurse assess the ability to abstract. The following paired objects are frequently used:

- Bicycle and bus
- Apple and pear
- Television and newspaper

A higher level reply would address function, whereas a description of structure would indicate more concrete thinking. To determine a patient's fund of general knowledge, the nurse can ask the patient to name the last five presidents, the mayor, five large cities, or the occupation of a well-known person.

> **NURSE ALERT.** The patient's educational level and any learning disabilities should be carefully evaluated. Mental retardation should be ruled out whenever possible.

Judgment

Judgment involves making decisions that are constructive and adaptive. It involves the ability to understand facts and draw conclusions from relationships.

Observations

Judgment can be evaluated by exploring the patient's involvement in activities, relationships, and vocational choices. For example, is the patient regularly involved in illegal or dangerous activities or frequently engaged in destructive relationships with others? It is also useful to determine if the judgments are deliberate or impulsive. Finally, several hypothetical situations can be presented for the patient to evaluate, such as the following:

1. What would you do if you found a stamped, addressed envelope lying on the ground?
2. How would you find your way out of a forest in the daytime?
3. What would you do if you entered your house and smelled gas?
4. If you won $10,000, what would you do with it?

NURSE ALERT.   Judgment is impaired in intoxicated patients and those with organic mental disorders, schizophrenia, psychotic disorders, and borderline or below average IQ. It may also be a problem for manic patients and those with personality disorders.

Insight

Insight refers to the patient's understanding of the nature of the illness.

Observations

The nurse must determine if the patient accepts or denies the presence of illness. In addition, the nurse should inquire if the patient blames the problem on someone else or some external factors. Several questions may help to determine the patient's degree of insight. What does the patient think about what the nurse has been told? What does the patient want others, including the nurse, to do about it?

NURSE ALERT. Impaired insight is associated with many psychiatric illnesses, including organic mental disorder, psychosis, substance abuse, eating disorders, personality disorders, and borderline IQ and below. Whether or not a patient sees the need for treatment also critically affects the therapeutic alliance, setting of mutual goals, implementation of the treatment plan, and future adherence to it.

Behavioral Rating Scales

A variety of behavioral rating scales and measurement tools are available as additional methods of assessment. Rating scales help clinicians perform the following:

1. Measure the extent of a patient's problems
2. Make an accurate diagnosis
3. Track patient progress over time
4. Document the efficacy of treatment

Frequently used scales include the following:

1. Beck Depression Inventory—self-reporting, 13-item scale designed to measure depth of depression and to screen depressed patients rapidly
2. Brief Psychiatric Rating Scale (BPRS)—clinician-administered, 18-item scale that provides rapid and efficient evaluation of treatment response by focusing on adult psychopathology
3. Clinical Global Impressions (CGI)—clinician-administered, three-item scale measuring severity of illness, global improvement, and efficacy of drug regimen
4. Hamilton Anxiety Scale (HAM-A)—clinician-administered, 14-item scale for patients with a diagnosis of anxiety
5. Hamilton Psychiatric Rating Scale for Depression (HAM-D)—clinician-administered, 21-item scale for assessing severity of an adult patient's depression and for showing changes in condition
6. Manic-State Rating Scale—clinician-administered, 26-item scale that measures manic symptoms, including frequency and intensity of behavior
7. Nurses' Observation Scale for Inpatient Evaluation (NOSIE)—30-item scale measuring patient behavior in adult

and geriatric wards, with nursing personnel providing measures of patients' strengths and pathological states

8. Self-Report Symptom Check List-90 (SCL-90)—self-reporting, 90-item scale that presents a list of problems and complaints and asks the patient how bothersome these problems, if present, have been during the past week

Sociocultural Context of Care

In each patient interaction, the psychiatric nurse should be aware of the broader world in which the patient lives. The nurse should realize that the patient's perception of health and illness, help-seeking behavior, and treatment adherence depends on the individual's unique beliefs, social norms, and cultural values. The culturally sensitive nurse understands the importance of social and cultural forces for the individual, recognizes the uniqueness of these aspects, respects nurse-patient differences, and incorporates sociocultural information into psychiatric nursing care.

Sociocultural Risk Factors

Sociocultural risk factors for psychiatric illness include the following:

1. Age
2. Ethnicity
3. Gender
4. Education
5. Income
6. Belief system

These predisposing factors can significantly increase the potential for developing a psychiatric disorder, decrease the potential for recovery, or both. No one or two of these factors alone can adequately describe the sociocultural context of psychiatric nursing care. Together, however, they provide a sociocultural profile of the patient that is essential to quality psychiatric nursing practice.

Sociocultural Stressors

Lack of awareness of these risk factors and their effect on the individual, along with lack of respect for sociocultural differences, can result in inadequate nursing care. Table 4-2 lists some

Table 4-2   Sociocultural stressors

Stressor	Definition
Disadvantagement	Lack of socioeconomic resources that are basic to biopsychosocial adaptation
Stereotype	Depersonalized conception of individuals within a group
Intolerance	Unwillingness to accept different opinions or beliefs from people of different backgrounds
Stigma	Attribute or trait deemed by the individual's social environment as different and diminishing
Prejudice	Preconceived, unfavorable belief about individuals or groups that disregards knowledge, thought, or reason
Discrimination	Differential treatment of individuals or groups not based on actual merit
Racism	Belief that inherent differences among the races determine individual achievement and that one race is superior

sociocultural stressors that also can hinder the quality of psychiatric care.

Sociocultural Assessment

Assessment of the patient's sociocultural risk factors and stressors greatly enhances the nurse's ability to establish a therapeutic alliance, identify the patient's problems, and develop a psychiatric nursing treatment plan that is accurate, appropriate, and culturally relevant. Box 4-5 presents questions that the nurse might ask related to each of the risk factors identified.

The psychotherapeutic treatment process also is influenced by the cultural and ethnic context of both the patient and the health-care provider. Together the nurse and patient need to agree on the nature of the patient's coping responses, the means for solving problems, and the expected outcomes of treatment.

Box 4-5   Questions Related to Sociocultural Risk Factors

Age

What is the patient's current stage of development?
What are the developmental tasks of the patient?
Are those tasks age-appropriate for the patient?
What are the patient's attitudes and beliefs regarding the specific age group?
With what age-related stressors is the patient currently coping?
What impact does the patient's age have on mental and physical health?

Ethnicity

What is the patient's ethnic background?
What is the patient's ethnic identity?
Is the patient traditional, bicultural, multicultural, or culturally alienated?
What are the patient's attitudes, beliefs, and values regarding the specific ethnic group?
With what ethnic-related stressors is the patient currently coping?
What impact does the person's ethnicity have on mental and physical health?

Gender

What is the patient's gender?
What is the patient's gender identity?
How does the patient define gender-specific roles?
What are the patient's attitudes and beliefs regarding males and females and masculinity and femininity?
With what gender-related stressors is the patient currently coping?
What impact does the person's gender have on mental and physical health?

Education

What is the patient's educational level?

Continued

Box 4-5   Questions Related to Sociocultural Risk Factors—cont'd

Education—cont'd

What were the patient's educational experiences like?

What are the patient's attitudes and beliefs regarding education in general and the patient's own education in particular?

With what education-related stressors is the patient currently coping?

What impact does the patient's education have on mental and physical health?

Income

What is the patient's income?

What is the source of the patient's income?

How does the patient describe the specific income group?

What are the patient's attitudes and beliefs regarding personal socioeconomic status?

With what economic-related stressors is the patient currently coping?

What impact does the patient's income have on mental and physical health?

Belief System

What are the patient's beliefs about health and illness?

What was the patient's religious or spiritual upbringing?

What are the patient's current religious or spiritual beliefs?

Who is the patient's regular health-care provider?

With what belief system–related stressors is the patient currently coping?

What impact does the patient's belief system have on mental and physical health?

your **INTERNET**
c o n n e c t i o n

NEUROSCIENCES ON THE INTERNET
http://www.lm.com/~nab
ERIC Clearinghouse on Assessment and Evaluation
http://ericAe2.EDUC.CUA.edu/main.htm
EthnoMed Ethnic Medicine Guide
http://www.hslib.washington.edu/clinical/ethnomed

Suggested readings

Comas-Diaz L, Greene B: *Women of color: integrating ethnic and gender identities in psychotherapy,* New York, 1994, The Guilford Press.

Dunner D: Diagnostic assessment, psychiatric assessment, *Psychiatric Clin N Am* 16:431, 1993.

Eisenberg L: The social construction of the human brain, *Am J Psychiatry* 152:1563, 1995.

Ellison J, Weinstein C, Hodel-Malinofsky T: *The psychotherapists guide to neuropsychiatry: Diagnostic and treatment issues,* Washington DC, 1994, American Psychiatric Press.

Gardner H: *Multiple intelligences,* New York, 1993, Basic Books.

Gaw A: *Culture, ethnicity, and mental illness,* Washington DC, American Psychiatric Press.

Gelfand D: *Aging and ethnicity,* New York, 1994, Springer Publishing Company.

Greenfield S: *The human mind explained: an owner's guide to the mysteries of the mind,* New York, 1996, Henry Holt and Company.

Brain imaging and psychiatry, *Harvard Mental Health Letter* 13:1, 1997.

Hayes A: Psychiatric nursing: what does biology have to do with it? *Arch Psychiatric Nurs* 9:216, 1995.

Hudak C, Gallo B: Quick review of neurodiagnostic testing, *Am J Nurs* 97:16cc, 1997.

Koslow S, et al: *The neuroscience of mental health, II: a report on neuroscience research,* US Dept of Health and Human Services, Public Health Service, NIH, NIMH, Rockville, MD, 1995.

LeDoux J: *The emotional brain: the mysterious underpinnings of emotional life,* New York, 1996, Simon & Shuster.

McCain N, Smith J: Stress and coping in the context of psychoimmunology: a holistic framework for nursing practice and research, *Arch Psychiatric Nurs* 8:221, 1994.

Morrison J: *The first interview: a guide for clinicians,* New York, 1993, The Guilford Press.

Roberts G, Leigh P, Weinberger D: *Neuropsychiatric disorders,* London, 1993, Wolfe.

Sederer L, Dickey B: *Outcomes assessment in clinical practice,* Baltimore, 1996, Williams and Wilkins.

Sommes-Flanagan J, Sommes-Flanagan R: *Foundations of therapeutic interviewing,* Boston, 1992, Allyn & Bacon.

Stuart G, Laraia M: *Principles and practice of psychiatric nursing,* ed 6, St Louis, 1998, Mosby.

Taggart S: *Living as if: belief systems in mental health practice,* San Francisco, 1994, Jossey-Bass Publishers.

Trzepacz P, Baker R: *The psychiatric mental status examination,* New York, 1993, Oxford University Press.

Environmental Context of Psychiatric Nursing Care

5

Managed Care

Managed care is a reality of the current health-care environment. In a well-functioning system of managed care a defined group of people receive treatment services that are clinically necessary and medically appropriate, have defined benefit parameters, are provided over a predetermined time, are in compliance with quality standards, and have anticipated and measurable outcomes. Currently the term *managed care,* as applied to mental and substance abuse disorders, has been replaced by *managed behavioral health care,* which refers to these disorders together as one set of health problems.

Defining Characteristics

Managed care differs significantly from the traditional fee-for-service health-care delivery system (Table 5-1). Managed care involves a major shift away from the person as customer to the *population* as customer. It deemphasizes high-cost, episodic, inpatient admissions and procedures in favor of creating a full continuum of care and then selecting the correct level of care and treatment setting. While the traditional system fostered duplication of services and technology among hospitals, managed care stimulates the consolidation of services, formation of networks, and use of primary care networks to provide both referral and gatekeeping activities.

Table 5-1 Comparison of traditional and managed care health delivery systems

Characteristic	Traditional System	Managed Care System
Provider focus	Specialized care of individual patient	Total care of member population
Pricing	Separate physician and hospital fee schedules	Discounts, case rates, capitation
Market share	Number of admissions Number of procedures Number of visits	Number of covered lives
Management focus	High inpatient occupancy rate	Low inpatient occupancy rate Correct level of care
Service line	Acute care programs as driving forces Inconsistent integration Physician dependent Individual services	Continuum of care Inpatient Partial hospitalization Outpatient Residential Home
Cost management	Payers assume admission rate risk Provider assumes length-of-stay risk	Provider networks assume all utilization risks Admission rate Length of stay

Costs	Cost per procedure Cost per hospitalization	Cost per life Inpatient days per 1000 Visits per 1000
Competition	Multiple hospitals for communities Duplication of services and technology	Increased consolidation and network formation as occupancy declines Closures Alternative uses of hospitals
Characteristic outcomes	Qualitative measures Reputation Facilities	Quantitative measures Quality Cost
Referral base	Focus on "high-tech" capabilities Separate physician and hospital "marketing" efforts	Ability to form primary care networks Mutual goals and strategies of providers and hospitals

---

Box 5-1   Types of Managed Care Plans

- **Health maintenance organizations (HMOs)** are organized delivery systems that provide care to a defined
  population, usually for a predetermined fixed
  amount (capitation rate). Consumers enrolled in HMOs
  are restricted to using HMO providers.
- **Preferred provider organizations (PPOs)** are plans that
  contract with a limited number of clinicians, most often
  physicians, and hospitals who provide care at discounted rates. Members of these plans are given
  financial incentives to use the "preferred providers"
  but are not prevented from using any provider of
  choice. Insurers or employers select the providers to
  be included in their preferred plan.
- **Point-of-service plans (POSs)** allow consumers to
  choose between delivery systems at the time they
  seek care. In a triple-option plan, for example,
  people can choose among an HMO, PPO, or fee-
  for-service plan. Financial incentives are usually
  provided to encourage people to use the least expensive option.

Managed care is not a single entity; rather, it can assume various types or forms (Box 5-1). The concept of *managed competition* is a purchasing strategy in which managed care organizations contract with several hospitals that provide cost-effective, comprehensive services. Consumers are then informed about the hospitals from which they may receive services, even though the facility may not be the patient's preferred choice.

Financial Aspects

A managed care system uses the following three major payment mechanisms:

1. *Discounted fee-for-service payment plan,* in which clinicians are paid for all services that have been authorized and provided to a consumer. The payment rate is discounted or is less than the clinician's standard fee schedule and often includes a provision for a copayment that must be collected from the consumer at each visit.

2. *Case rate system,* in which the clinician is paid a flat fee for a predefined episode of care. The most well-known case rate system is Medicare's Diagnostic Related Groups (DRGs), in which Medicare pays a flat fee for a particular hospitalization episode regardless of how many days the person was hospitalized. This system shifts the financial risk to the provider because the provider receives a flat fee regardless of the actual cost of care.

3. *Capitation system,* in which the consumer pays a fixed fee—a per member, per month (PMPM) premium. In return the managed care company that receives the PMPM fee agrees to provide all the medically necessary health care required by all the covered customers in the group. In this case, most of the financial risk lies with the managed care company, who must deliver all necessary health care within the premiums received by their population pool. HMOs are the best-known examples of capitated payment systems.

Managed care exerts cost control measures in the following ways:

- *Preadmission certification* takes into account the patient's medical and psychiatric status, level of functioning, socioenvironmental factors, and procedural issues associated with treatment. The managed care reviewer's role is to determine the most appropriate form of treatment and the proper treatment setting. In this way the reviewer acts as a gatekeeper on issues of cost and quality.

- *Utilization review* evaluates the appropriateness and necessity of services and procedures. It is a way of monitoring the care and services administered and has the most immediate impact on patient care. The patient's treatment plan, diagnostic and therapeutic interventions, and discharge planning are continuously monitored by a third party. This third party determines reimbursement for treatment based on current standards of care. The review and approval can be done before providing the services *(precertification review),* at the time the service is rendered *(concurrent review),* or after the service has been provided *(retrospective review),* which may be used retroactively to deny payment.

- *Case management* typically is targeted to those patients who have treatment complications, have high-expense episodes of care, or need alternative, less expensive treatments or settings.

This group often includes patients with serious and persistent mental illness. Case management focuses on achieving desirable patient outcomes, appropriate lengths of stay, efficient use of resources, and patient involvement and satisfaction.

Clinical Impact

The changing mental health-care environment is impacting practice issues for psychiatric nurses in several important ways.

Access to Services

Access can be defined as the degree to which services and information about care are conveniently and easily obtained. It is an important part of any effective mental health-care delivery system. Today more than half the people who seek health care for mental disorders are treated by primary care practitioners. However, many who appear to need care do not receive it, either from a primary care or specialty provider. When access to mental health care is made difficult, the overall costs of general medical care increase because those with behavioral health-care problems are high-level users of medical services. An ideal comprehensive health-care system would (1) provide multiple points of entry for treatment, including direct access through self-referral, (2) adequately fund behavioral health-care benefits and services, (3) reimburse all types of providers for their services, and (4) find ways of measuring and reinforcing standards for the accessibility, appropriateness, quality, and effectiveness of treatment.

Treatment Parity

Many people who need treatment for mental illnesses and chemical dependency disorders do not receive it because their insurance policies deny or restrict coverage for such treatment. A law passed by the U.S. Congress in 1996 ended the cash benefits and Medicare and Medicaid coverage for persons whose disability is based on drug addiction or alcoholism. Also in 1996, treatment parity (equality) legislation was passed in several states, and a national mental health parity bill in the United States was passed with the following provisions:

- Calls for parity in all health insurance for lifetime and annual limits between physical and mental illness (excluding alcohol and substance abuse) if a plan provides mental health benefits at all (plans are not required to provide such benefits)

- Excludes businesses with fewer than 56 employees from the requirement
- Is effective Jan. 1, 1998

Clinical Appropriateness

Clinical appropriateness refers to the degree to which the type, amount, and level of clinical services are delivered to promote the most positive clinical outcomes for the consumer. To meet managed care's criteria of clinical appropriateness, behavioral health-care organizations are developing diversified but fully integrated continuums of care by expanding their own services, contracting with other health-care organizations, or affiliating with area providers. These continuums of care must be capable of providing services and alternative levels of care to children, adolescents, adults, and elderly people requiring either psychiatric or substance abuse services. The goal is to provide "one-stop shopping" for managed behavioral care consumers and to secure market dominance in a particular geographical area. Box 5-2 lists the range of services expected in an integrated continuum of care in behavioral health.

Practice Guidelines

Practice guidelines in psychiatric care are strategies for mental health-care delivery developed to facilitate clinical decision making

---

Box 5-2   Services in Integrated Behavioral Continuum of Care

---

Traditional Services
- 24-hour emergency assessment
- Inpatient services
- Structured outpatient care
- Medication evaluation and management
- Individual and group therapy

Expanded Services
- Crisis intervention program
- Outpatient services—group and individual
- Intensive outpatient programs
- Partial hospitalization or day treatment

Continued

Box 5-2   Services in Integrated Behavioral Continuum of Care—cont'd

Expanded Services—cont'd

- In-home services
- Residential services
- Aftercare services
- Psychoeducational programs

New Product Lines

- 23-hour holding beds
- Crisis stabilization units
- Mobile evaluation teams
- In-home crisis stabilization and treatment
- Group home services
- Triaging and referral services
- Structured outpatient programs
- In-home therapy
- Family therapy
- Marital therapy
- Crisis resolution therapy
- Intensive short-term outpatient therapy
- Therapeutic wilderness program
- Therapeutic foster care

and to provide patients with critical information concerning their different treatment options. The goals of practice guidelines are as follows:

- Document preferred or "best" practices.
- Increase consistency in care.
- Facilitate outcome research.
- Enhance the quality of care provided.
- Improve staff productivity.
- Reduce costs.

Practice guidelines are identified by various terms, such as clinical protocols, practice parameters, and treatment standards. Guidelines have been developed by professional associations such as the American Psychiatric Association (Box 5-3), by managed care companies, and by academic centers using techniques such as expert consensus and data analysis.

Box 5-3   Practice Guidelines Developed by the American Psychiatric Association

- Eating disorders (February 1993)
- Major depressive disorder (April 1993)
- Bipolar disorder (December 1994)
- Substance use disorders (November 1995)
- Psychiatric evaluation (November 1995)
- Nicotine dependence (October 1996)
- Schizophrenia (April 1997)
- Alzheimer's disease (May 1997)
- Panic disorder and related anxiety disorders (November 1997*)
- Delirium (March 1998*)
- Geriatric care (March 1998*)
- Mental retardation (March 1998*)

*Anticipated publication date.

Clinical Pathways

A clinical pathway identifies the key clinical processes and corresponding timelines to which the patient must adhere to achieve standard outcomes within a specified time. It is a written plan that serves as a map and timetable for the efficient, effective delivery of health care. Valid clinical pathways are developed over time by a multidisciplinary team. They can be constructed around diagnoses from the *Diagnostic and Statistical Manual of Mental Disorders,* fourth edition (DSM-IV), North American Nursing Diagnosis Association (NANDA) diagnoses, clinical conditions, treatment stages, clinical interventions, or targeted behaviors. They are most often used in inpatient settings, serve as a shortened version of the multidisciplinary plan of care for a patient, and require close team cooperation and monitoring of ongoing quality improvement. Some clinical settings have computerized their pathways to enhance the consistency and efficiency of care provided.

The key elements of the clinical pathway are (1) identifying a target population; (2) describing the expected outcome of treatment in a measurable, realistic, and patient-centered way; (3) specifying treatment strategies and interventions; and (4) documenting patient care activities, variances, and goal achievement. Fig. 5-1 presents

STAGE OF TREATMENT	CRISIS ← - - - →	ACUTE ← - - - →
GOAL	STABILIZATION	REMISSION
TREATMENT FOCUS	High-risk behaviors	Symptoms and coping responses
ASSESSMENTS	Risk factor assessment Nursing assessment	Nursing assessment Medical assessment Supplemental scales
EXPECTED OUTCOME	NO HARM TO SELF OR OTHERS	SYMPTOM RELIEF
Consults		
Tests/labs		
Symptom management		
Medications		
Treatments		
Activity		
Safety		
Teaching		
Nutrition		
Discharge planning		

Figure 5-1
General clinical pathway template for psychiatric care.

MAINTENANCE ◄ - - - ►	HEALTH PROMOTION
RECOVERY	OPTIMAL LEVEL OF WELLNESS
Functional status	Quality of life
Functional status scale	Well-being scale
IMPROVED FUNCTIONING	OPTIMAL QUALITY OF LIFE

Figure 5-1—cont'd
For legend see opposite page.

an example of the format of a general clinical pathway for psychiatric treatment through the four stages of the care continuum. Any one stage of psychiatric treatment (crisis, acute, maintenance, or health promotion) identified in this clinical pathway can be singled out and developed in detail. At this time, great variability exists in the format and use of clinical pathways in psychiatric care.

Outcomes Measurement

Outcomes are the extent to which services are cost effective and have a favorable effect on the consumer's symptoms, functioning, and well-being. Outcomes include all those factors affecting the patient and family while they are involved in the health care system, such as health status, functional status, quality of life, presence or absence of illness, type of coping response, and satisfaction with treatment. Outcome evaluation can focus on a clinical condition, an intervention, or a caregiving process. The variety of outcomes that can be examined include clinical, functional, satisfaction, and financial indicators related to the provision of psychiatric care (Box 5-4). The specific purposes of outcomes measurement are as follows:

- Evaluate the outcomes of care
- Suggest changes in treatment
- Evaluate program effectiveness
- Profile the practice pattern of providers
- Determine the most appropriate level of care

Box 5-4 Categories of Outcome Indicators

Clinical Outcome Indicators
- High-risk behaviors
- Symptomatology
- Coping responses
- Relapse
- Recurrence
- Readmission
- Number of treatment episodes
- Medical complications
- Incidence reports
- Mortality

Box 5-4   Categories of Outcome Indicators—cont'd

Functional Outcome Indicators
- Functional status
- Social interaction
- Activities of daily living
- Occupational abilities
- Quality of life
- Family relationships
- Housing arrangement

Satisfaction Outcome Indicators

Patient/family satisfaction with:
- Outcomes
- Providers
- Delivery system
- Caregiving process
- Organization

Financial Outcome Indicators
- Cost per treatment episode
- Revenue per treatment episode
- Length of inpatient stay
- Use of health-care resources
- Costs related to disability

- Predict the path of a patient's illness and recovery
- Contribute to quality improvement programs

Accountability Issues

Driven by the demand to demonstrate quality and reduce costs, the behavioral health-care environment is confronted by new issues of accountability.

Patients' Rights

With managed care it is clear that individuals will have limits placed on their choice of providers, service settings, and sometimes even treatment options. If limited options are available, patients may be unable to take advantage of newer treatments that may help them. Partly in response to these concerns, the Center for Mental Health Services has developed a set of principles that emphasizes the need for comprehensive services, continuity of care, and responsiveness to the needs of service recipients. The principles cover the areas of quality of care, consumer participation, accessibility, affordability, linkages and integration, and accountability.

Provider Concerns

Providers are increasingly aware of their responsibility to provide cost-effective care within an environment of shrinking psychiatric resources. New dilemmas arise for clinicians who must balance a responsibility to both an individual patient and a population of patients. Also, managed care has increased the tension between patient advocacy and resource allocation, because providers may feel the need to serve the organization's "bottom line" and thus may jeopardize the individual patient's interests.

When mental health clinicians become part of networks or organized systems of care, they become subject to the review of others. Their activities are often routinely measured, and they are held accountable for the type and amount of care they deliver. Many mental health professionals view this negatively, but others see it as a positive trend leading to an overall improvement in behavioral health-care services.

Providers also struggle with (1) the ambiguity of many of the rules, regulations, and expectations of this new health-care environment; (2) the overreliance of managed care on treatment protocols that diminish professional judgment and minimize individual patient or clinical factors; and (3) the reduced clinician productivity resulting from administrative burdens and excessive documentation. Finally, providers' roles and functions are often subject to confusion, and the realities of the new environment often escalate conflict among the mental health disciplines rather than enhance interdisciplinary collaboration.

Service Settings

Mental health facilities have been criticized for denying inpatient care or transferring patients to another facility for economic reasons when it is not in the patient's best interests. Another effect of managed care has been the recent layoffs and downsizing of inpatient facilities because of decreased inpatient census and increased managed competition. The resulting shortage of staff and the increased work the remaining members are asked to assume may adversely affect the care provided. In addition, while staffing is decreasing, acuity of inpatient disorders is increasing, which more urgently demands an adequate number of well-trained staff to deliver quality patient care.

Another challenge to service setting accountability arises with information management. Computerized patient records are providing standardized formats for easier data collection and analyses. Clinical, financial, and administrative information systems are being integrated to measure outcomes related to quality and costs of care. Important accountability issues are related to confidentiality, appropriate uses of data, and protection of data, particularly in an area as sensitive as psychiatric and substance abuse disorders.

Accrediting Organizations

Accrediting organizations for managed care include the Utilization Review Accreditation Committee (URAC), the Joint Commission on Accreditation of Healthcare Organizations (JCAHO), and the National Committee on Quality Assurance (NCQA). NCQA is an independent, nonprofit HMO-accrediting organization composed of independent health-care quality experts, employers, labor union officials, and consumers. In 1991 NCQA adopted standards that assess performance in the following six areas:

1. Quality improvement and information
2. Utilization management
3. Credentialing of providers
4. Members' rights and responsibilities
5. Preventive health services
6. Medical records

NCQA accreditation is designed for most managed care companies. NCQA has the longest performance record in managed care accreditation, and its accreditation is mandated by law in many states.

Nursing Roles in Managed Care

Nurses bring great assets to the managed care arena through their rich blend of skills and expertise. Although nursing activity varies greatly based on education, experience, certification, service setting, and geographical location, psychiatric nurses have assumed many roles in managed care, including the following:

- Mental health clinician
- Case manager
- Evaluation and triage nurse
- Utilization review nurse
- Patient educator
- Risk manager
- Quality improvement officer
- Marketing and development specialist
- Corporate manager

Throughout all the changes in the mental health-care environment, individuals, families, and communities continue to experience significant emotional problems. Thus the need for psychiatric nurses, as competent and caring professionals, will also continue. Nurses must be proactive, however, in realigning their positions within the changing environment. As hospitals downsize, more nurses will be needed in community and home settings. Many of the programs needed by patients in the community have not yet been designed. Psychiatric nurses can assume a leadership role in this new frontier.

your **INTERNET** c o n n e c t i o n

Association of Managed Care Providers
http://www.comed.com/amcp/intro.html
Institute for Behavioral Health Care
http://www.ibh.com/

Suggested readings

Boyle P, Callahan D: Managed care in mental health: the ethical issues, *Health Aff* 14:8, 1995.

Chrisman A: How kids are different: child and adolescent services under managed care, *J Pract Psychiatry Behav Health* 3:236, 1996.

Corcoran K, Vandiver V: *Maneuvering the maze of managed care: skills for mental health practitioners,* New York, 1996, Free Press.

Goodman M, Brown J, Deitz P: *Managing managed care II: a handbook for mental health professionals,* Washington DC, 1996, American Psychiatric Press.

Hogan M: Managing the whole system of care, *New Dir Ment Health Serv* 72:13, 1996.

Hoyt M: *Brief therapy and managed care,* San Francisco, 1995, Jossey-Bass.

Institute of Medicine: *Managing managed care: quality improvement in behavioral health,* Washington DC, 1997, National Academy Press.

Kashner T, Rush A, Altshuler K: Managed care and the focus on outcomes research, *J Pract Psychiatry Behav Health* 3:135, 1997.

Mandersheid R, Henderson M: *Federal and state legislative and program directions for managed care: implications for case management,* Rockville, Md, 1995, Center for Mental Health Services.

McDaniel C, Erlen J: Ethics and mental health service delivery under managed care, *Issues Ment Health Nurs* 17:11, 1996.

Mitchell A, Reaghard D: Managed care and psychiatric–mental health nursing services: implications of practice, *Issues Ment Health Nurs* 17:1, 1996.

Olsen D: Ethical considerations of managed care in mental health treatment, *J Psychosoc Nurs* 32:25, 1996.

Sederer L, Bennett M: Managed mental health care in the United States: a status report, *Admin Policy Ment Health* 23:289, 1996.

Sederer L, Dickey B: *Outcomes assessment in clinical practice,* Baltimore, 1996, Williams & Wilkins.

Smith G et al: Principles for assessment of patient outcomes in mental health care, *Psychiatric Serv* 48:1033, 1997.

Strosahl K: Mind and body primary mental health care: new model for integrated services, *Behav Healthcare Tomorrow* 4:96, 1996.

Trabin T, Freeman M: *Managed behavioral healthcare,* Tiburon, Calif, 1995, Centralink.

Tusaie-Mumfrod K, Hahn C: Practical outcome evaluation: patient behavioral health care demonstration project, *Issues Ment Health Nurs* 17:59, 1996.

Ziglin A: *Confidentiality and the appropriate uses of data,* Rockville, Md, 1995, US Department of Health and Human Services, SAMSHA.

Legal-Ethical Context of Psychiatric Nursing Care

6

The practice of psychiatric nursing is influenced by the law, particularly regarding the rights of patients and the quality of their care. Many of the laws vary from state to state, and nurses are required to become familiar with the legal provisions of their own state. Knowledge of the law enhances the freedom of both the nurse and the patient.

Hospitalization and Community Treatment

The process of hospitalization can be traumatic or supportive, depending on the institution, attitude of family and friends, response of the staff, and type of admission. Table 6-1 presents characteristics that distinguish between the two types of admission to psychiatric hospitals: voluntary and involuntary.

Involuntary Admission (Commitment)

The legal basis for involuntary confinement is either the police power of the state for the protection of society or *parens patriae,* the state's duty to protect citizens who cannot protect themselves. Fig. 6-1 lists common procedural elements of the commitment process. Action is begun with a petition by a relative, friend, public official, physician, or any interested citizen stating that the person is mentally ill and in need of treatment. An examination of the patient's mental status is then completed by one or two physicians.

Table 6-1   Characteristics of the two types of admission to psychiatric hospitals

	Voluntary Admission	Involuntary Admission
Admission	Written application by patient	Application did not originate with patient
Discharge	Initiated by patient	Initiated by hospital or court but not by patient
Status of civil rights	Retained in full by patient	Patient may retain none, some, or all, depending on state law
Justification	Voluntarily seeks help	Mentally ill and one or more of the following: 1. Dangerous to self or others 2. Need for treatment 3. Unable to meet own basic needs

The decision as to whether the patient requires hospitalization is then made, and who decides this determines the nature of the commitment. Medical certification means that physicians make the decision. Court or judicial commitment is decided by a judge or jury in a formal hearing. The patient may retain legal counsel to prepare for the hearing. Administrative commitment is determined by a special tribunal of hearing officers.

If the individual is determined to be (1) dangerous to self or others, (2) mentally ill and in need of treatment, and/or (3) unable to meet basic needs such as food and shelter, that person is hospitalized.

Discharge

Voluntary patients of lawful age may initiate their own discharge. Most states require that patients give written notice of their desire for discharge. For patients who are leaving against medical advice, most hospitals request they sign a form stating this. If voluntary patients elope from the hospital, they can be brought back only if

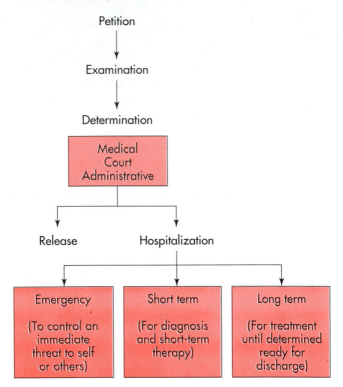

Figure 6-1
Diagram of the involuntary commitment process.

they again voluntarily agree. If they refuse to return to the hospital, they must be discharged or involuntary commitment procedures must be initiated. Involuntary patients have lost the right to leave the hospital when they wish. If a committed patient elopes from the hospital, the staff has the legal obligation to notify the police and committing courts.

Involuntary Community Treatment

Involuntary community treatment can be provided for those in need through (1) outpatient commitment, (2) preventive commitment, and (3) conditional release from the hospital. These initiatives arose from the mandate to offer psychiatric patients treatment in the least restrictive setting.

Outpatient commitment is the process by which the courts can order patients "committed" to a course of outpatient treatment specified by their clinicians. This type of commitment provides an alternative to inpatient treatment for those who meet the involuntary commitment criterion of dangerousness to self or others.

Preventive commitment permits commitment for outpatients who do not yet meet the usual commitment criteria but will do so soon without intervention. The criteria used for preventive commitment are sometimes referred to as a *predicted deterioration standard.* In this case a person is believed to need treatment to prevent a relapse, which would likely result in the individual becoming imminently dangerous.

Conditional release involves continued supervision of a person who has been released from the hospital. The hospital or court informs the person of the conditions for release, such as reporting to a medication clinic. Violation of these conditions usually results in rehospitalization. This approach is used primarily to determine if the individual is able to function in the community under supervision.

These initiatives are alternatives to address the pressing problem of the homeless but nondangerous mentally ill individual who is in need of psychiatric treatment and stabilization in the community. They may be most beneficial for revolving-door patients—those who stop taking their medication shortly after discharge, rapidly deteriorate, and soon require rehospitalization.

Ethical Considerations

All nurses must analyze their beliefs regarding voluntary and involuntary hospitalization and community treatment of psychiatric patients. Psychiatric nurses, patients, families, and citizens need to address such issues as the value of commitment, goals of hospitalization, treatment received while hospitalized, community alternatives, and quality of life. Nurses are responsible for reviewing commitment procedures in their state and working for the necessary clinical, ethical, and legal reform.

Patients' Rights

Box 6-1 lists patients' rights that have been adopted by many states. Some of these rights especially important to psychiatric nurses are discussed next.

Box 6-1   Rights of Psychiatric Patients

- Right to communicate with people outside the hospital through correspondence, telephone, and personal visits
- Right to keep clothing and personal effects with them in the hospital, except for potentially dangerous objects
- Right to religious freedom
- Right to be employed, if possible
- Right to manage and dispose of property
- Right to execute wills
- Right to enter into contractual relationships
- Right to make purchases
- Right to education
- Right to habeas corpus
- Right to independent psychiatric examination
- Right to civil service status
- Right to retain licenses, privileges, or permits established by law, such as a driver's or professional license
- Right to sue or be sued
- Right to marry and divorce
- Right not to be subject to unnecessary mechanical restraints
- Right to periodic review of status
- Right to legal representation
- Right to privacy
- Right to informed consent
- Right to treatment
- Right to refuse treatment
- Right to treatment in the least restrictive setting

Right to communicate with people outside the hospital. The patient is free to visit and hold telephone conversations in privacy and send unopened letters to anyone.

Right to personal effects. The patient has the right to bring a limited amount of personal items. This does not hold the hospital responsible for their safety, however, and does not relieve the hospital staff of ensuring the patient's safety.

Right to execute wills. A person's competency to make a will is known as "testamentary capacity." Persons can make a valid will if they (1) know that they are making a will, (2) know the nature and extent of their property, and (3) know who their friends and relatives are and what the relationship means. Each of these criteria must be met and documented for the will to be considered valid.

Right to habeas corpus. All patients retain this right, which allows for a court of law to require the speedy release of individuals who can show they are being deprived of their liberty and detained illegally.

Right to independent psychiatric examination. The patient may demand a psychiatric examination by a physician of choice. If this physician determines that the patient is not mentally ill, the person must be released.

Right to privacy. The individual may keep some personal information completely secret from others.

Confidentiality allows the disclosure of certain information to another person, but this is limited to strictly authorized individuals. *Privileged communication* is a legal phrase that applies only in court-related proceedings. It means that the listener cannot disclose information from an individual unless the speaker gives permission. Privileged communication does not apply to hospital charts, and most states do not provide for privileged communication between nurses and patients. In addition, therapists have the responsibility to breach the confidentiality of the relationship to warn a potential victim of impending violence by a patient.

Right to informed consent. A physician must explain the treatment to the patient, including its possible complications, side effects, and risks. The physician must obtain the patient's consent, which must be competent, understanding, and voluntary. Box 6-2 lists the reasonable information to be disclosed in obtaining informed consent.

Right to treatment. Criteria for adequate treatment are defined in three areas: (1) a humane psychological and physical environment, (2) a qualified staff with a sufficient number of members to administer treatment, and (3) individualized treatment plans.

Right to refuse treatment. Patients may refuse treatment unless they have been legally determined to be incompetent. A determination of *incompetency* requires that the person has a mental disorder resulting in a defect in judgment and that this defect makes this person incapable of handling personal affairs. Incompetency can only be reversed through another court hearing.

Box 6-2   Obtaining Informed Consent

INFORMATION TO DISCLOSE

- **Diagnosis:** description of patient's problem
- **Treatment:** nature and purpose of proposed treatment
- **Consequences:** risks and benefits of proposed treatment, including physical and psychological effects, costs, and potential problems
- **Alternatives:** viable alternatives to proposed treatment and their risks and benefits
- **Prognosis:** expected outcome with treatment, with alternative treatments, and without treatment

PRINCIPLES OF INFORMING

- Assess patient's ability to give informed consent.
- Simplify the language so that laypersons can understand.
- Offer opportunities for patient and family to ask questions.
- Test patient's understanding after the explanation.
- Reeducate as often as needed.
- Document all relevant factors, including what was disclosed; patient's understanding, competency, and voluntary agreement to treatment; and the actual consent.

Ethical Considerations

Ensuring patients' rights is often complicated by ethical considerations that the nurse must carefully examine. Many ethical dilemmas arise from health care professionals' "paternalistic" attitude toward their patients, which reduces adult patients to the status of children and interferes with their freedom of action. Ethical questions can also arise for the psychiatric nurse in implementing patients' rights, such as the right to treatment, right to refuse treatment, and right to treatment in the least restrictive setting. All nurses participate in some therapeutic psychiatric regimens with ambiguous scientific and ethical bases. Thus each nurse must analyze such ethical dilemmas as freedom of choice versus coercion, helping versus imposing values, and focusing on cure versus prevention. Nurses assume an active role in defining adequate treatment and deciding important resource allocations for mentally ill patients.

Legislative Initiatives

Other legislation has also changed the nature of psychiatric care and service delivery in the United States.

Protection and Advocacy Act

Under the Protection and Advocacy for Mentally Ill Individuals Act of 1986, all states must designate an agency that is responsible for protecting the rights of mentally ill patients. The following three areas of advocacy would help to maximize the fulfillment of patients' rights:

1. To educate the mental health staff and to implement policies and procedures that recognize and protect patients' rights
2. To establish an additional procedure to permit the speedy resolution of problems, questions, or disagreements that occur based on legal rights
3. To provide access to legal services when patients' rights have been denied

Americans with Disabilities Act

The Americans with Disabilities Act (ADA), passed in 1990, protects more than 43 million Americans with one or more physical or mental disabilities from discrimination in jobs, public services, and accommodations. It prohibits discrimination against people with physical and mental disabilities in hiring, firing, training, compensation, and advancement in employment. Employers are prohibited from asking job applicants whether they have a disability, and medical examinations and questions about disability may be required only if the concerns are job related and necessary.

Advanced Directives

Advanced directives came about as a result of the Patient Self-Determination Act (PSDA) of 1990. Written while a person is competent, these documents specify how decisions about treatment should be made if the person were to become incompetent. Use of advanced directives seems particularly appropriate for persons with mental illness who may alternate between periods of competence

Table 6-2   Three sets of criteria typically used to determine criminal responsibilities of a mentally ill offender

Name of Test	Criteria
M'Naghten rule	1. The individual did not know the nature and quality of the act. 2. The individual did not know that the act was wrong.
Irresistable impulse test	An individual is impulsively driven to commit the criminal act with lack of premeditation and a strong urge to do so. This test is seldom used without other criteria.
American Law Institute's test	An individual lacks the capacity to "appreciate" the wrongfulness of the act or to "conform" conduct to the requirements of the law. It excludes the psychopath and is a popular criterion for determining criminal responsibility.

and incompetence. They could, for example, formalize a patient's wishes about forced medication or treatment setting.

Psychiatry and Criminal Responsibility

Three sets of criteria are used in the United States to determine the criminal responsibility of an offender with a mental illness (Table 6-2). Of these, the American Law Institute's test (ALI) is the most frequently used. The two types of insanity defense are as follows:

1. Not guilty by reason of insanity (NGBI)
2. Guilty but mentally ill (GBMI)

Both outcomes typically result in the hospitalization of patients in state mental hospitals or treatment facilities provided in the penal institution.

Legal Role of the Nurse

The psychiatric nurse has rights and responsibilities attendant to each of three legal roles: nurse as provider, nurse as employee, and nurse as citizen. Nurses may experience a conflict of interest among these rights and responsibilities. Professional nursing judgment requires a careful examination of the context of nursing care, the possible consequences of nursing actions, and the feasible alternatives the nurse might employ.

Malpractice

Malpractice involves the failure of a professional person to provide the type of care given by members of the person's profession in the community, resulting in harm to the patient. Most malpractice claims are filed under the law of negligent tort. A *tort* is a civil wrong for which the injured party is entitled to compensation. Under the law of negligent tort the plaintiff must prove the following:

1. A legal duty of care existed.
2. The nurse performed the duty negligently.
3. Damages were incurred by the patient as a result.
4. The damages were substantial.

your **INTERNET**
c o n n e c t i o n

Bazelon Center for Mental Health Law
http://www.bazelon.org/
Medical-Legal Consulting Institute, Inc.
http://ourworld.compuserve.com/homepages/
Medical_Legal_Consulting

Suggested readings

Appelbaum P: *Almost a revolution: mental health law and the limits of change,* New York, 1994, Oxford University Press.

Appelbaum P: Managed care and the next generation of mental health law, *Psychiatric Serv* 47:27, 1996.

Benedek E: Emerging issues in forensic psychiatry: from the clinic to the courthouse, *New Direct Mental Health Serv* 69, 1996.

Forensic nursing, *J Psychosoc Nurs Ment Health Serv* 31, 1993.

Galen K: Assessing psychiatric patients' competency to agree to treatment plans, *Hosp Community Psychiatry* 44:361, 1993.

Group for the Advancement of Psychiatry: *Forced into treatment: the role of coercion in clinical practice,* Washington, DC, 1994, American Psychiatric Press.

Haas L, Malouf J: *Keeping up the good work: a practitioner's guide to mental health ethics,* ed 2, Sarasota, FL, 1995, Professional Resource Press.

Joseph-Kinzelman A et al: Clients' perceptions of involuntary hospitalization, *J Psychosoc Nurs* 32:28, 1994.

Lucksted A, Coursey R: Consumer perceptions of pressure and force in psychiatric treatments, *Psychiatr Serv* 46:146, 1995.

Munetz M et al: The effectiveness of outpatient civil commitment, *Psychiatr Serv* 47:1251, 1996.

Sabin J: What confidentiality standards should we advocate for in mental health care, and how should we do it? *Psychiatric Services* 48:35, 1997.

Schauer C: Special report: protection and advocacy: what nurses need to know, *Archives of Psychiatric Nursing* 9:233, 1995.

Simon R: *Psychiatry and law for clinicians,* Washington, DC, 1992, American Psychiatric Association.

Slovenko R: *Psychiatry and criminal culpability,* New York, 1995, Wiley & Sons.

Smith C: Use of involuntary outpatient commitment in community care of the seriously and persistently mentally ill patient, *Issues Ment Health Nurs* 16:275, 1995.

Smith S: Liability and mental health services, *Am J Orthopsychiatry* 64:235, 1994.

Stuart G, Laraia M: *Principles and practice of psychiatric nursing,* ed 6, St Louis, 1998, Mosby.

Sundram C: Implementation and activities of protection and advocacy programs for persons with mental illness, *Psychiatr Serv* 46:702, 1995.

Trudeau M: Informed consent: the patient's right to decide, *J Psychosoc Nurs Ment Health Serv* 31:9, 1993.

Wasserbauer L: Mental illness and the Americans with disabilities act: understanding the fundamentals, *J Psychosocial Nursing* 35:22, 1997.

Wright E, Pescosolido B, Penslar R: New ethical challenges to mental health services research in the era of community-based care, *J Mental Health Admin* 24:140, 1997.

Implementing Clinical Practice Standards

7

Nursing Defined

The American Nurses' Association (ANA) defines nursing as "the diagnosis and treatment of human responses to actual or potential health problems."[1] This definition suggests the following four defining characteristics of nursing[1]:

1. *Phenomena*—range of health-related responses observed in sick and well people that are the focus of nursing diagnosis and treatment
2. *Theory*—concepts, principles, and processes that guide nursing intervention and understanding of health-related responses
3. *Actions*—interventions to prevent illness and promote health
4. *Effects*—evaluation of nursing actions in relation to identified health responses and anticipated outcome of nursing care

Standards of Psychiatric–Mental Health Clinical Nursing Practice

Standards of Psychiatric–Mental Health Clinical Nursing Practice[2] describes a competent level of professional nursing care and professional performance common to nurses engaged in psychiatric–mental health nursing practice in any setting. These standards apply to nurses who are qualified by education and experience to practice at either the basic level or the advanced level of

123

psychiatric–mental health nursing. Because some nursing activities depend greatly on variables such as patient situation, clinical setting, and instances of individual judgment, language such as "as appropriate," "when possible," and "as applicable" is used to recognize circumstances where exceptions may occur.

Standards of Care*

Standards of care pertain to professional nursing activities demonstrated by the nurse throughout the nursing process. These involve assessment, nursing diagnosis, outcome identification, planning, implementation, and evaluation. The nursing process is the foundation of clinical decision making and encompasses all significant action taken by nurses in providing psychiatric–mental health care to all patients.

Fig. 7-1 outlines the nursing conditions and nursing behaviors related to each of the psychiatric nursing standards of care.

Standard I. Assessment

The psychiatric–mental health nurse collects client health data.

RATIONALE

The assessment interview—which requires linguistically and culturally effective communication skills, interviewing, behavior observation, database record review, and comprehensive assessment of the client and relevant systems—enables the psychiatric–mental health nurse to make sound clinical judgments and plan appropriate interventions with the client.

Standard II. Diagnosis

The psychiatric–mental health nurse analyzes the assessment data in determining the diagnoses.

RATIONALE

The basis for providing psychiatric–mental health nursing care is the recognition and identification of patterns of response to actual or potential psychiatric illnesses and mental health problems.

---

* Reprinted with permission from American Nurses' Association: *A statement of psychiatric–mental health clinical nursing practice and standards of psychiatric–mental health clinical nursing practice,* Washington, DC, 1994, The Association.

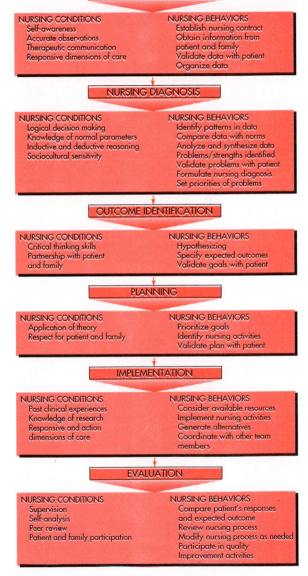

ASSESS

NURSING CONDITIONS
Self-awareness
Accurate observations
Therapeutic communication
Responsive dimensions of care

NURSING BEHAVIORS
Establish nursing contract
Obtain information from
patient and family
Validate data with patient
Organize data

NURSING DIAGNOSIS

NURSING CONDITIONS
Logical decision making
Knowledge of normal parameters
Inductive and deductive reasoning
Sociocultural sensitivity

NURSING BEHAVIORS
Identify patterns in data
Compare data with norms
Analyze and synthesize data
Problems/strengths identified
Validate problems with patient
Formulate nursing diagnosis
Set priorities of problems

OUTCOME IDENTIFICATION

NURSING CONDITIONS
Critical thinking skills
Partnership with patient
and family

NURSING BEHAVIORS
Hypothesizing
Specify expected outcomes
Validate goals with patient

PLANNING

NURSING CONDITIONS
Application of theory
Respect for patient and family

NURSING BEHAVIORS
Prioritize goals
Identify nursing activities
Validate plan with patient

IMPLEMENTATION

NURSING CONDITIONS
Past clinical experiences
Knowledge of research
Responsive and action
dimensions of care

NURSING BEHAVIORS
Consider available resources
Implement nursing activities
Generate alternatives
Coordinate with other team
members

EVALUATION

NURSING CONDITIONS
Supervision
Self-analysis
Peer review
Patient and family participation

NURSING BEHAVIORS
Compare patient's responses
and expected outcome
Review nursing process
Modify nursing process as needed
Participate in quality
Improvement activities

Figure 7-1
The nursing conditions and behaviors related to the psychiatric nursing standards of care.

Standard III. Outcome identification

The psychiatric–mental health nurse identifies expected outcomes individualized to the client.

RATIONALE

Within the context of providing nursing care, the ultimate goal is to influence health outcomes and improve the client's health status.

Standard IV. Planning

The psychiatric–mental health nurse develops a plan of care that prescribes interventions to attain expected outcomes.

RATIONALE

A plan of care is used to guide therapeutic intervention systematically and achieve the expected client outcomes.

Standard V. Implementation

The psychiatric–mental health nurse implements the interventions identified in the plan of care.

RATIONALE

In implementing the plan of care, psychiatric–mental health nurses use a wide range of interventions designed to prevent mental and physical illness and promote, maintain, and restore mental and physical health. Psychiatric–mental health nurses select interventions according to their level of practice. At the basic level the nurse may select counseling, milieu therapy, self-care activities, psychobiological interventions, health teaching, case management, health promotion and health maintenance, and a variety of other approaches to meet the mental health needs of clients. In addition to the intervention options available to the basic-level psychiatric–mental health nurse, at the advanced level the certified specialist may provide consultation, engage in psychotherapy, and prescribe pharmacological agents where permitted by state statutes or regulations.

Standard Va. Counseling

The psychiatric–mental health nurse uses counseling interventions to assist clients in improving or regaining their previous coping abilities, fostering mental health, and preventing mental illness and disability.

Standard Vb. Milieu therapy

The psychiatric–mental health nurse provides, structures, and maintains a therapeutic environment in collaboration with the client and other health-care providers.

Standard Vc. Self-care activities

The psychiatric–mental health nurse structures interventions around the client's activities of daily living to foster self-care and mental and physical well-being.

Standard Vd. Psychobiological interventions

The psychiatric–mental health nurse uses knowledge of psycho-biological interventions and applies clinical skills to restore the client's health and prevent further disability.

Standard Ve. Health teaching

The psychiatric–mental health nurse, through health teaching, assists clients in achieving satisfying, productive, and healthy patterns of living.

Standard Vf. Case management

The psychiatric–mental health nurse provides case management to coordinate comprehensive health services and ensure continuity of care.

Standard Vg. Health promotion and health maintenance

The psychiatric–mental health nurse employs strategies and interventions to promote and maintain mental health and prevent mental illness.

Advanced Practice interventions Vh-Vj

The following interventions (Vh-Vj) may be performed only by the certified specialist in psychiatric–mental health nursing.

Standard Vh. Psychotherapy

The certified specialist in psychiatric–mental health nursing uses individual, group, and family psychotherapy, child psychother-apy, and other therapeutic treatments to assist clients in foster-ing mental health, preventing mental illness and disability, and improving or regaining previous health status and functional abilities.

Standard Vi. Prescription of pharmacological agents

The certified specialist uses prescription of pharmacological agents, in accordance with the state nursing practice act, to treat symptoms of psychiatric illness and improve functional health status.

Standard Vj. Consultation

The certified specialist provides consultation to health-care providers and others to influence the plans of care for clients and to enhance the abilities of others to provide psychiatric and mental health care and effect change in systems.

Standard Vl. Evaluation

The psychiatric–mental health nurse evaluates the client's progress in attaining expected outcomes.

RATIONALE

Nursing care is a dynamic process involving change in the client's health status over time, giving rise to the need for new data, different diagnoses, and modifications in the plan of care. Therefore evaluation is a continuous process of appraising the effect of nursing interventions and the treatment regimen on the client's health status and expected health outcomes.

Standards of Professional Performance*

Standards of professional performance describe a competent level of behavior in the professional nursing role, including activities related to quality of care, performance appraisal, education, collegiality, ethics, collaboration, research, and resource utilization. All psychiatric–mental health nurses are expected to engage in professional role activities appropriate to their education, position, and practice setting. Therefore standards or measurement criteria are used to identify these activities.

Standard I. Quality of care

The psychiatric–mental health nurse systematically evaluates the quality of care and effectiveness of psychiatric–mental health nursing practice.

---

* Reprinted with permission from American Nurses' Association: *A statement on psychiatric–mental health clinical nursing practice and standards of psychiatric–mental health clinical nursing practice,* Washington, DC, 1994, The Association.

RATIONALE

The dynamic nature of the mental health-care environment and the growing body of psychiatric nursing knowledge and research provide both the impetus and the means for the psychiatric–mental health nurse to be competent in clinical practice, to continue to develop professionally and to improve the quality of client care.

Standard II. Performance appraisal

The psychiatric–mental health nurse evaluates own psychiatric–mental health nursing practice in relation to professional practice standards and relevant statutes and regulations.

RATIONALE

The psychiatric–mental health nurse is accountable to the public for providing competent clinical care and has an inherent responsibility as a professional to evaluate the role and performance of psychiatric–mental health nursing practice according to standards established by the profession and regulatory bodies.

Standard III. Education

The psychiatric–mental health nurse acquires and maintains current knowledge in nursing practice.

RATIONALE

The rapid expansion of knowledge pertaining to basic and behavioral sciences, technology, information systems, and research requires a commitment to learning throughout the psychiatric–mental health nurse's professional career. Formal education, continuing education, certification, and experiential learning are some of the means the psychiatric–mental health nurse uses to enhance nursing expertise and advance the profession.

Standard IV. Collegiality

The psychiatric–mental health nurse contributes to the professional development of peers, colleagues, and others.

RATIONALE

The psychiatric–mental health nurse is responsible for sharing knowledge, research, and clinical information with colleagues, through formal and informal teaching methods, to enhance professional growth.

Standard V. Ethics

The psychiatric–mental health nurse's decisions and actions on behalf of clients are determined in an ethical manner.

RATIONALE

The public's trust and its right to humane psychiatric–mental health care are upheld by professional nursing practice. The foundation of psychiatric–mental health nursing practice is the development of a therapeutic relationship with the client. The psychiatric–mental health nurse engages in therapeutic interactions and relationships that promote and support the healing process. Boundaries need to be established to safeguard the client's well-being and to prevent the development of intimate or sexual relationships.

Standard VI. Collaboration

The psychiatric–mental health nurse collaborates with the client, significant others, and health-care providers in providing care.

RATIONALE

Psychiatric–mental health nursing practice requires a coordinated, ongoing interaction between consumers and providers to deliver comprehensive services to the client and the community. Through the collaborative process, different abilities of health-care providers are used to solve problems, communicate, and plan, implement, and evaluate mental health services.

Standard VII. Research

The psychiatric–mental health nurse contributes to nursing and mental health through the use of research.

RATIONALE

Nurses in psychiatric–mental health nursing are responsible for contributing to the further development of the field of mental health by participating in research. At the basic level of practice the psychiatric–mental health nurse uses research findings to improve clinical care and identifies clinical problems for research study. At the advanced level the psychiatric–mental health nurse engages and/or collaborates with others in the research process to discover, examine, and test knowledge, theories, and creative approaches to practice.

Standard VIII. Resource utilization

The psychiatric–mental health nurse considers factors related to safety, effectiveness, and cost in planning and delivering client care.

RATIONALE

The client is entitled to psychiatric–mental health care that is safe, effective, and affordable. As the cost of health care increases, treatment decisions must be made in such a way as to maximize resources and maintain quality of care. The psychiatric–mental health nurse seeks to provide cost-effective quality care by using the most appropriate resources and delegating care to the most appropriate, qualified health-care provider.

your **INTERNET**
c o n n e c t i o n

American Nurses Association: NURSING WORLD
http://www.ana.org
Canadian Nurses Association
http://www.cna-nurses.ca

References

1. American Nurses' Association: *Nursing: a social policy statement,* Kansas City, Mo, 1980, The Association.
2. American Nurses' Association: *A statement on psychiatric–mental health clinical nursing practice and standards of psychiatric–mental health clinical nursing practice,* Washington, DC, 1994, The Association.

Suggested readings

American Psychiatric Association: Practice guidelines for psychiatric evaluation of adults, *Am J Psychiatry* 152(suppl):67, 1995.

Artnak K, Dimmitt J: Choosing a framework for ethical analysis in advanced practice settings: the case for casuistry, *Arch Psychiatr Nurs* 10:16, 1996.

Burdick M, Stuart G, Lewis L: Measuring nursing outcomes in a psychiatric setting, *Iss Mental Health Nurs* 15:137, 1994.

Dombeck M, Brody S: Clinical supervision: a three-way mirror, *Arch Psychiatr Nurs* 9:3, 1995.

Eppard J, Anderson J: Emergency psychiatric assessment: the nurse, psychiatrist, and counselor roles during the process, *J Psychosoc Nurs* 33:17, 1995.

Farkas-Cameron M: Clinical supervision in psychiatric nursing, *J Psychosoc Nurs* 33:31, 1995.

Grohol J: *The insider's guide to mental health resources online,* New York, 1997, The Guilford Press.

Gross D, Fogg L, Conrad B: Designing interventions in psychosocial research, *Arch Psychiatr Nurs* 7:259, 1993.

Guide to behavior resources on the Internet: a review of mental health and substance abuse web sites, mailing lists, and support forums, New York, 1997, Faulkner & Grau, Inc.

Hastings C: Perspectives in ambulatory care: the changing multidisciplinary team, *Nurs Econ* 15:106, 1997.

Keller G: Management for quality: continuous quality improvement to increase access to outpatient mental health services, *Psychiatric Serv* 48:821, 1997.

Kobak K: Computer-administered symptom rating scales, *Psychiatric Serv* 47:367, 1996.

Kobak K et al: Computerized screening for psychiatric disorders in an outpatient community mental health clinic, *Psychiatric Serv* 48:1048, 1997.

Krch-Cole E et al: Bridging the chasm: incorporating the medically compromised patient into psychiatric practice, *J Psychosoc Nurs* 35:28, 1997.

Lieberman H, Goldberg F, Kaplin G: The CD-ROM as a multipurpose clinical and management tool, *Psychiatric Serv* 48:1014, 1997.

Lim R: The Internet: applications for mental health clinicians in clinical settings, training and research, *Psychiatr Serv* 47:597, 1996.

Merwin E, Mauck A: Psychiatric nursing outcome research: the state of the science, *Arch Psychiatr Nurs* 9:311, 1995.

Moch S et al: Linking research and practice through discussion, *Image* 29:189, 1997.

Poster E, Dee V, Randell B: The Johnson Behavioral Systems Model as a framework for patient outcome evaluation, *J Am Psychiatric Nurs Assoc* 3:73, 1997.

Price J, Stevens H, LaBarre M: Spiritual caregiving in nursing practice, *J Psychosoc Nurs* 33:6, 1995.

Redman B: *The process of patient teaching,* St Louis, 1993, Mosby.

Stuart G, Laraia M: *Principles and practice of psychiatric nursing,* ed 6, St Louis, 1998, Mosby.

Walters J, Neugeboren B: Collaboration between mental health organizations and religious institutions, *Psychiatric Rehab J* 19:51, 1995.

Weaver R et al: Computerized treatment planning, *Hosp Com Psychiatry* 45:825, 1994.

Wilson J, Hobbs H: Therapeutic partnership: a model for clinical practice, *J Psychosoc Nurs* 33:27, 1995.

Continuum of Psychiatric Care

8

Psychiatric nurses provide treatment throughout the continuum of care. This includes interventions related to primary, secondary, and tertiary prevention.

Primary Prevention

Primary prevention is biological, social, or psychological intervention that promotes health and well-being or reduces the *incidence* of illness in a community by altering the causative factors before they can do harm.

Assessment of Preventive Nursing Needs

Assessment of a patient's need for preventive nursing measures includes identification of the following:

1. A stressor that precipitates maladaptive responses
2. A target or vulnerable population group that is at high risk in relation to the stressor, including children and adolescents, new families, families experiencing divorce or illness, women, and elderly persons

Planning and Implementation

A national incentive has been undertaken to promote health and prevent disease in the United States. Specific nursing interventions in primary prevention include health education, environmental change, and support of social systems.

Health education

Health education involves strengthening individuals and groups through building competence. The assumption is that many maladaptive responses result from a lack of competence. This involves a lack of perceived control over one's life, a lack of effective coping strategies, and the resulting lowered self-esteem. Health education has the following four levels of intervention:

1. Increasing the individual's or group's awareness of issues and events related to health and illness, such as normal developmental tasks
2. Increasing one's understanding of the dimensions of potential stressors, possible outcomes (both adaptive and maladaptive), and alternative coping responses
3. Increasing one's knowledge of where and how to acquire the needed resources
4. Increasing the individual's or group's problem-solving skills, interpersonal skills, tolerance of stress and frustration, motivation, hope, and self-esteem

Environmental change

Preventive interventions may be made to modify the individual's or group's immediate environment or the larger social system. These interventions are particularly helpful when the environment has placed new demands on the patient, does not respond to developmental needs, and provides little positive reinforcement. Environmental changes may include the following types:

1. *Economic*—allocating resources for financial aid or assistance in budgeting and managing income
2. *Work*—receiving vocational testing, guidance, education, or retraining that can result in new jobs or careers
3. *Housing*—moving to new quarters, which may mean leaving or returning to family and friends; improving existing housing; gaining or losing family, friends, or roommates
4. *Family*—attending child care facilities, nursery school, grade school, or camp; obtaining access to recreational, social, religious, or community services
5. *Political*—influencing health-care structures and procedures; participating in community planning and development; addressing legislative issues

Support of social systems

Strengthening social supports is a way of buffering or cushioning the effects of a potentially stressful event. The following four types of preventive intervention are possible:

1. Assess communities and neighborhoods to identify problem areas and high-risk groups.

2. Improve linkages between community support systems and formal mental health services.
3. Strengthen existing caregiving networks, including church groups, civic organizations, women's groups, work and neighborhood supports, and self-help groups.
4. Help the individual or group develop, maintain, expand, and use the existing social network.

Evaluation

The nurse should consider the following points in evaluating primary prevention interventions or programs:

1. *Efficacy.* Does the program or intervention do more good than harm in the opinion of its proponents?
2. *Effectiveness.* Does the intervention do more good than harm to its target population?
3. *Efficiency.* Is the intervention being made available to those who could benefit from it? Is there optimum use of resources?
4. *Length and timing.* Does any evidence indicate the optimum length or timing of the intervention program?
5. *Harmful effects.* Are there data to suggest that the interventions may have harmful effects (e.g., unfavorable consequences of labeling)?
6. *Screening programs.* Is there any information about the program's sensitivity, specificity, and predictive accuracy?
7. *Possible high-risk groups.* Does any evidence suggest that the program would be more efficient if it applied to a specific population at increased risk?
8. *Economic analysis.* What are the results of the cost-benefit and cost-effectiveness analyses?

Secondary Prevention

Secondary prevention involves reducing the *prevalence* of a disorder. Secondary prevention activities include early case finding, screening, and prompt effective treatment. Crisis intervention is an important secondary prevention treatment modality.

Crisis

A crisis is an internal disturbance that results from a stressful event or a perceived threat to the self. A person's usual repertoire of coping mechanisms becomes ineffective in dealing with the threat, and the person experiences a state of disequilibrium and a rise in anxiety. The threat, or precipitating event, can usually be identified.

The goal of crisis intervention is for the person to return to the precrisis level of functioning. Crises are self-limited in time, and the intense conflict they represent can be a period of increased vulnerability, which can stimulate personal growth. What the person does with the crisis will determine whether growth or disorganization results.

Balancing factors

In describing the resolution of a crisis, some important balancing factors need to be considered (Fig. 8-1).

Successful resolution of the crisis is more likely if the individual's perception of the event is realistic rather than distorted, if situational supports are available so that others can help solve the problem, and if coping mechanisms are available to help alleviate anxiety.

Types of crises

1. *Maturational crises.* These are transitional or developmental periods in a person's life during which psychological equilibrium is upset, such as during adolescence, parenthood, marriage, or retirement. Maturational crises require role changes. The nature and extent of the maturational crises can be influenced by the adequacy of role models, interpersonal resources, and the ease of others in accepting the new role.
2. *Situational crises.* These occur when a specific external event upsets an individual's psychological equilibrium or a group's equilibrium. Examples include the loss of a job, divorce, death, school problems, and illness.
3. *Adventitious crises.* These are accidental, uncommon, and unexpected crises that may result in multiple losses and gross environmental changes, such as through fires, floods, nuclear accidents, and mass tragedies. They do not occur in the lives of everyone, but when they do occur, they cause severe stress and challenge all of a person's coping abilities.

Table 8-1 presents the five phases of human disaster response.

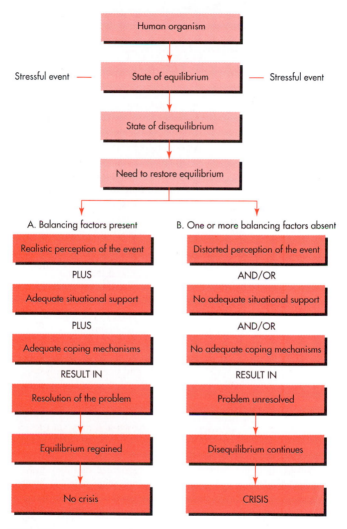

Figure 8-1
Effect of balancing factors in a stressful event.
From Aguilera DC: *Crisis intervention: theory and methodology,* ed 8, St Louis, 1998, Mosby.

Table 8-1 Five phases of human disaster response

Phase	Response
Impact	This phase includes the event itself and is characterized by shock, panic, or extreme fear. The person's judgment and assessment of reality factors are very poor, and self-destructive behavior may be seen.
Heroic	A cooperative spirit exists between friends, neighbors, and emergency teams. Constructive activity at this time can help to overcome feelings of anxiety and depression, but overactivity can lead to "burnout."
Honeymoon	This phase begins to appear 1 week to several months after the disaster. The need to help others is sustained, and the money, resources, and support received from various agencies help to renew the community. Psychological and behavioral problems may be overlooked.
Disillusionment	This phase lasts from about 2 months to 1 year and is a time of disappointment, resentment, frustration, and anger. Victims often begin to compare their neighbors' plights with their own and may start to resent, envy, or show hostility toward others.
Reconstruction and reorganization	Individuals recognize that they must come to grips with their own problems. They begin to rebuild their homes, businesses, and lives. This phase may last for years after the disaster.

Data from Frederick C, Garrison J: *Behav Today* 12:32, 1981.

Assessment

During the assessment phase the nurse must obtain data regarding the nature of the crisis and its effect. The nurse should make the following specific assessments:

1. *Identify the precipitating event,* including the needs that are threatened by the event and the point at which symptoms appeared.
2. *Identify the person's perception of the event,* including the underlying themes and memories associated with the event.
3. *Identify the nature and strength of the person's support system and coping resources,* including family, friends, and significant others who might be of help.
4. *Identify the person's previous strengths and coping mechanisms,* including successful and unsuccessful coping strategies.

Planning and Implementation

Dynamics underlying the crisis are formulated, alternative solutions to the problem are explored, and steps for achieving the solutions are designated. This process is described in the Patient Education Plan for coping with crisis on p. 140-141. *The expected outcome of nursing care is that the patient will recover from the crisis event and return to a precrisis level of functioning.* A more ambitious expected outcome would be for the patient to recover from the crisis event and attain a higher than precrisis level of functioning with improved quality of life. Four levels of crisis intervention exist, representing a hierarchy from the most basic (level 1) to the most in-depth (level 4):

1. *Environmental manipulation.* These interventions directly change the person's physical or interpersonal situation for the purpose of providing situational support or removing stress.
2. *General support.* This provides individuals with the feeling that the nurse is on their side and will help them. The nurse's demonstration of warmth, acceptance, empathy, and caring results in this type of support.
3. *Generic approach.* This type of crisis intervention is designed to reach individuals at high risk and people in great numbers as soon as possible. It applies a specific

Patient Education Plan
Coping with Crisis

Content	Instructional Activities	Evaluation
Describe the crisis event.	Ask about the details of the crisis event, including: 1. A timeline of the crisis event 2. Who was affected 3. The events of the crisis 4. Any precipitating events Determine precrisis level of functioning. Discuss patient's perception of the crisis. Determine acute and long-term needs, threats, and challenges.	Patient describes the crisis event in full detail. Patient discusses precrisis level of functioning and perceptions of the crisis. Patient's needs are identified.
Explore feelings, thoughts, and behaviors related to the crisis event.		

Identify coping mechanisms.	Ask how stressful events have been handled in the past. Analyze whether these approaches are adaptive or maladaptive for the current crisis event. Suggest additional coping strategies.	Patient identifies adaptive coping mechanisms for the current crisis event.
Develop a plan for coping adaptively with the crisis event.	Reinforce adaptive coping mechanisms and health defenses. With patient, construct a coping plan specific for the aftermath of the crisis event.	Patient develops a plan for coping with the crisis event.
Assign patient activities from the coping plan.	Review implementation of the coping plan. Help patient generalize coping strategies for use in future crisis events.	Patient reports satisfaction with coping abilities and level of functioning.

method to all people facing a similar crisis, such as assisting disaster victims to work through the grieving process.

4. *Individual approach.* This approach involves the diagnosis and treatment of a specific problem in a specific patient. The individual approach is effective with all types of crises and in a combination of crises or when homicidal or suicidal risk exists.

The techniques of crisis intervention are active, focal, and explorative. They are not interpretive because the goal is quick resolution of an immediate problem. Table 8-2 summarizes crisis intervention techniques. Table 8-3 describes interventions for working with individuals and families with stress resulting from crises.

Evaluation

1. Has the person returned to the precrisis level of functioning?
2. Have the person's original needs, which were threatened by the precipitating or stressful event, been met?
3. Have the person's maladaptive behaviors or symptoms subsided?
4. Have the person's adaptive coping mechanisms begun to function again?
5. Does the person have a strong support system on which to rely?
6. What has the person learned from this experience that may be helpful in coping with future crises?

Tertiary Prevention

Tertiary prevention activities attempt to reduce the severity of a disorder and its associated *disability*.

Rehabilitation

Rehabilitation is the process of enabling individuals to return to the highest possible level of functioning. Psychiatric rehabilitation developed from a need to create opportunities for people diagnosed with severe mental illness to live, learn, and work in community environments of their choice. Rehabilitation proposes that those with mental illnesses should be perceived as people

Table 8-2   Techniques of crisis intervention

Technique	Definition	Example
Abreaction	Ventilation of feelings that takes place as patients verbally recount emotionally charged areas	"Tell me about how you have been feeling since you lost your job."
Clarification	When the nurse encourages patients to express more clearly the relationship between certain events in their life	"I've noticed that after you have an argument with your husband, you become sick and can't leave your bed."
Suggestion	Process of influencing individuals so that they accept an idea or belief, particularly the belief that the nurse can help them feel better	"Many other people have found it helpful to talk about this, and I think you will, too."
Manipulation	Use of patients' emotions, wishes, or values to their benefit in the therapeutic process	"You seem to be very committed to your marriage, and I think you will work through these issues and have a stronger relationship in the end."
Reinforcement of behavior	Giving patients positive responses to adaptive behavior	"That's the first time you were able to defend yourself with your boss, and it went very well. I'm so pleased that you were able to do it."

Continued

Table 8-2   Techniques of crisis intervention—cont'd

Technique	Definition	Example
Support of defenses	Encouragement of the use of defenses that result in adaptive gratification and the discouragement of those that result in maladaptive gratification	"Going for a bicycle ride when you were so angry was very helpful, since when you returned, you and your wife were able to talk things through."
Raising self-esteem	Helping patients to regain feelings of self-worth	"You are a very strong person to be able to manage the family all this time. I think you will be able to handle this situation, too."
Exploration of solutions	Examination of alternative modes of action geared toward solving the immediate problem	"You seem to know many people in the computer field. Couldn't you contact some of them to see if they might know of available jobs?"

Table 8-3 Nursing interventions for crisis events

Target Areas	Nursing Interventions
Basic needs	Provide liaison to social agencies.
Physical deficits	Attend to physical emergencies.
	Refer to other health-care providers as necessary.
Psychological effects	
Shock	Listen attentively to the crisis details.
Confusion	Give nurturing support; permit regression.
Denial	Permit intermittent denial; identify patient's primary concern.
Anxiety	Provide structure; enact antianxiety interventions.
Lethargy/heroics	Encourage sublimation and constructive activity.
Protective factors	
Coping	Encourage patient's favored, adaptive coping mechanisms; emphasize rationalization, humor, and sublimation.
Self-efficacy	Support patient's previous successes and belief in own abilities; dilute irrational self-doubts; emphasize power of expectations to produce results.
Support	Add social supports to patient's world; provide professional support; refer for counseling when necessary; help patient generalize new coping strategies.

Modified from Hardin SB: In McBride AB, Austin JK, editors: *Psychiatric–mental health nursing: integrating the behavioral and biological sciences,* Philadelphia, 1996, WB Saunders.

with disabilities. Similar to those with physical disabilities, people with psychiatric disabilities need a wide range of services, often for extended periods. Psychiatric rehabilitation uses a person-centered, people-to-people approach that differs from the traditional medical model of care (Table 8-4).

Table 8-4   Comparison of psychiatric rehabilitation and traditional medical model of care

Psychiatric Rehabilitation	Traditional Medical Model
Focus on wellness and health, not symptoms	Focus on disease/illness and symptoms
Based on patient's abilities and functional behavior	Based on patient's disabilities and intrapsychic functioning
Caregiving in natural settings	Treatment in institutional settings
Adult-to-adult relationship	Expert-to-patient relationship
Minimal medications used; minor symptoms tolerated	Medications used until symptoms controlled
Case management in partnership with patient	Decision making and treatment choice by physician
Emphasis on strengths, self-help, and interdependence	Emphasis on dependence and compliance

Assessment of Rehabilitative Nursing Needs

The individual

1. Identification of the nature and intensity of stressors
2. Exploration of the other advantages the patient experiences by being disabled (secondary gain)
3. Identification of coping resources
4. Assessment of community living skills (Table 8-5)

The family

1. Analysis of the family structure, including developmental stage, roles, responsibilities, norms, and values
2. Exploration of family attitudes toward the mentally ill member
3. Analysis of the emotional climate around the family
4. Identification of the social supports available to the family, including extended family, friends, financial support, religious involvement, and community contacts
5. Identification of the family's understanding of the patient's problem and the plan of care

Table 8-6 describes the categories and definitions of support needs expressed by family caregivers.

Table 8-5   Potential skilled activities needed to achieve goal of psychiatric rehabilitation

Physical	Emotional	Intellectual
Living Skills		
Personal hygiene	Human relations	Money management
Physical fitness	Self-control	Use of community resources
Use of public transportation	Selective reward	Goal setting
Cooking	Stigma reduction	Problem development
Shopping	Problem solving	
Cleaning	Conversational skills	
Sports participation		
Using recreational facilities		
Learning Skills		
Being quiet	Speech making	Reading
Paying attention	Question asking	Writing
Staying seated	Volunteering answers	Arithmetic
Observing	Following directions	Study skills
Punctuality	Asking for directions	Hobby activities
	Listening	Typing
Working Skills		
Punctuality	Job interviewing	Job qualifying
Use of job tools	Job decision making	Job seeking
Job strength	Human relations	Specific job tasks
Job transportation	Self-control	
Specific job tasks	Job keeping	
	Specific job tasks	

From Anthony WA: *Principles of psychiatric rehabilitation,* Baltimore, 1980, University Park Press.

Table 8-6   Categories and definitions of support needs expressed by family caregivers

Emotional Support Categories

Acceptance	Absence of stigmatization; acceptance of caregiver despite being related to a mentally ill patient
Commitment	Demonstrating to caregiver a commitment to patient's well-being; sharing the burden of caregiving, if only through contact with caregiver
Social involvement	Social contacts and companionship for caregiver
Affective	Showing caring and love for caregiver, including concern for well-being (with qualities of sympathy, compassion, and occasionally empathy)
Mutuality	Reciprocity in supportive exchanges

Feedback Support Categories

Affirmation	Validation of actions, feelings, and decisions associated with caregiving role
Listening	Active listening by support person; providing a "sounding board"; allowing for unburdening by caregiver
Talking	Opportunity to talk with another person (without the quality of active listening, emotional presence, or the feeling of unburdening)

Informational or Cognitive Support Categories

Illness information	Information about patient's illness, care, or supervision
Behavior management	Information about behavior management strategies
Coping	Advice about personal coping strategies for caregiver
Decision making	Help in decision-making process regarding caregiving issues; offering solutions
Perspective	Supportive interactions that give caregiver a new perspective about caregiving or about caregiving situation

Instrumental Support Categories

Resources	Help in locating resources, negotiating systems, or advocating for needs
Respite	Providing time off for caregiver and support for meeting caregiver's needs
Care/help	Providing help with actual tasks of caregiving, including physical care assistance and monitoring activities (watching patient's behavior and setting limits)
Backup	Help available when needed, including financial help
Household	Help with such home activities as repairs, grocery shopping, or housecleaning

From Norbeck J, Chafetz L, Skodol-Wilson H, Weiss SJ: *Nurs Res* 40:208, 1991.

The community

1. Assessment of existing community agencies that provide services to mentally ill people and their families
2. Identification of gaps in available services or in the effectiveness of existing services

Table 8-7 describes the services needed by patients with serious and persistent mental illness.

Planning and Implementation

The individual

1. Mutually determine realistic nurse-patient goals based on the patient's nursing diagnoses.
2. Focus on fostering independence by maximizing the patient's strengths and potential.
3. Facilitate referrals to alternative care programs that assist the patient to function independently or interdependently in the community; may be psychosocial rehabilitation programs or community support programs.
4. Assist the patient to become involved in a social skills training program that uses cognitive and behavioral techniques.
5. Identify resistances to change, if any, and assist the patient to overcome the resistance or find acceptable alternatives.
6. Teach the patient about relevant health-care needs, including physical health and mental health. A Patient Education Plan for psychiatric patients in rehabilitation programs is presented on pp. 154 and 155.
7. Act as the patient's advocate in dealing with significant others and community agencies.
8. Assist the patient to develop a reliable social support network.

The family

1. Establish a partnership with the family with the goal of assisting the patient.
2. Provide the patient and family with psychoeducation about the mental illness and the coping skills that will assist with successful community living (Box 8-1).
3. Provide the family with feedback on the effectiveness of their interactions.

Text continued on p. 156

Table 8-7   Comprehensive array of services and opportunities for patients with serious mental illness

Basic Needs and Opportunities	Special Needs and Opportunities
Shelter	**General Medical Services**
Protected (with health, rehabilitative, or social services provided on site)	Physician assessment and care
Hospital	Nursing assessment and care
Nursing home	Dentist assessment and care
Intermediate care facility	Physical and occupational therapy
Crisis facility	Speech and hearing therapy
Semiindependent (linked to services)	Nutrition counseling
Family home	Medication counseling
Group home	Home health services
Cooperative apartment	
Foster care home	**Mental Health Services**
Emergency housing facility	Acute treatment services
Other board and care home	Crisis stabilization
Independent (access to services)	Diagnosis and assessment
Apartment	Medication monitoring (psychoactive)
Home	Self-medication training
	Psychotherapies
	Hospitalization: acute and long-term care

Continued

Table 8-7   Comprehensive array of services and opportunities for patients with serious mental illness—cont'd

Basic Needs and Opportunities	Special Needs and Opportunities
Food, Clothing, and Household Management	**Habilitation and Rehabilitation**
Fully provided meals	Social and recreational skills development
Food purchase and preparation assistance	Life skills development
Access to food stamps	Leisure time activities
Homemaker service	
	Vocational
Income or Financial Support	Prevocational assessment counseling
Access to entitlements	Sheltered work opportunities
Employment	Transitional employment
	Job development and placement

Meaningful Activities

Work opportunities
Recreation
Education
Religious and spiritual
Human and social interaction

Integrative Services

Patient identification and outreach
Individual assessment and service planning
Case service and resource management
Advocacy and community organization
Community information
Education and support

Social Services

Family support
Community support assistance
Housing and milieu management
Legal services
Entitlement assistance

From Department of Health and Human Services Steering Committee on the Chronically Mentally Ill: *Toward a national plan for the chronically mentally ill*, Pub No (ADM)81-1077, Washington, DC, 1981, US Government Printing Office.

Patient Education Plan
Coping with Psychiatric Illness

Content	Instructional activities	Evaluation
Identify and describe common psychiatric diagnoses.	Provide handouts outlining behaviors. Discuss coping behaviors. Assign homework from lay literature. Compare mental illness to physical illness.	Patient recognizes characteristics of the diagnosis. Patient distinguishes between cure and coping.
Describe the role of stress in contributing to psychiatric disorders.	Sensitize patient to signs of increased stress. Define stress as a test of coping skills. Teach relaxation exercises.	Patient verbalizes level of stress. Patient performs relaxation exercises and describes a reduction in perceived stress.
Assist to gain a sense of control by recognizing personal pattern of signs and symptoms.	Provide feedback when symptomatic behavior occurs. Instruct patient to keep a diary of behaviors and to identify symptoms.	Patient consistently labels symptoms and seeks professional help when necessary.

Assist in development of social skills to enable participation in vocational and recreational activities.	Role-play social interaction in a variety of situations. Plan field trips to community activities. Arrange supervised vocational training in real work settings.	Patient participates in progressively more independent social and work activities.
Identify and describe community support systems.	Provide a list of community support programs, including self-help groups, mental health care agencies, and social agencies. Invite representatives of programs to speak to patient group. Escort to first agency contact.	Patient selects community programs that offer needed resources. Patient is able to access agency independently.
Describe and discuss psychoactive medications.	Instruct about actions, side effects, and contraindications to common psychoactive medications. Distribute handouts describing patient's medications. Suggest systems to help patient remember when to take medication and how much.	Patient describes characteristics of prescribed medications. Patient reports effects of prescribed medications. Patient takes medication as prescribed.

Modified from Buckwalter KC, Kerfoot KM: *J Psychosoc Nurs Ment Health Serv* 20:15, 1982.

Box 8-1   Elements of a Plan for Psychoeducation

- Signs and symptoms
- Natural course of the illness
- Possible etiologies
- Diagnostic tests and measures
- Indicated lifestyle changes
- Treatment options
- Expected treatment outcomes
- Medication effects and side effects
- Therapeutic strategies
- Adaptive coping responses
- Potential compliance problems
- Early warning signs of relapse
- Balancing needs and taking care of self

---

4. Refer the family for formal family therapy, if needed.
5. Refer the family to a self-help group.
6. Assist the family to find respite care services.
7. Provide the family with information on available crisis intervention services.

The community

1. Provide education about mental health and mental illness to community groups.
2. Participate in community advocacy groups to encourage the development of comprehensive mental health services.
3. Foster the development of collaborative networks among community groups involved in or advocating mental health services.
4. Be aware of and involved in the political process at the local, state, and national levels.

Evaluation

Program evaluation

1. Individual program evaluation may include the following:
   - Cost effectiveness
   - Licensure status
   - Accomplishment of stated objectives

- Patient outcomes
- Patient or staff satisfaction
2. Commonalities among a group of programs may also be assessed.
3. Programs may be evaluated at a systems level for relevance to community needs and resource utilization.

Patient evaluation

1. The needs and levels of functioning of individual patients tend to change over time. The nurse must consider this when evaluating patient progress.
2. Evaluation criteria for individual patients must be based on the individual's behavior and treatment goals. Criteria that have been identified for evaluation of patient response to rehabilitation programs include the following:
   - Involvement in community activities, including rehabilitation programs
   - Hospitalization recidivism rates
   - Ability to find and maintain employment

your **INTERNET**
c o n n e c t i o n

NAMI:
National Alliance for the Mentally Ill
http://www.nami.org
A Consumer's Guide to Mental Health Information
http://www.iComm.ca/madmagic/help/help.html

Suggested readings

Aguilera D: *Crisis intervention: theory and methodology,* ed 8, St Louis, 1998, Mosby.

Bauer M, McBride L: Psychoeducation: conceptual framework and practical considerations, *J Pract Psychiatry Behav Health* 3:18, 1997.

Biegel D, Song L, Milligan S: A comparative analysis of family caregivers' perceived relationships with mental health professionals, *Psychiatr Serv* 46:477, 1995.

Blumenkrantz D: *Fulfilling the promise of children's services: why primary prevention efforts fail and how they can succeed,* San Francisco, 1992, Jossey-Bass.

Byre C et al: Wellness education for individuals with chronic mental illness living in the community, *Iss Mental Health Nurs* 15:239, 1994.

Cohen S et al: Stages of nursing's political development: where we've been and where we ought to go, *Nurs Outlook* 44:259, 1996.

Corrigan P, Garman A: Considerations for research on consumer empowerment and psychosocial interventions, *Psychiatric Serv* 48:347, 1997.

Fisher D: Health care reform based on an empowerment model of recovery by people with psychiatric disabilities, *Hosp Comm Psychiatry* 45:913, 1994.

Francell E: My role as a consumer-provider: challenges and opportunities, *J Psychosoc Nurs* 34:29, 1996.

Freedy J, Hobfoll S: *Traumatic stress: from theory to practice,* New York, 1995, Plenum.

Hatfield A, Lefley H: *Surviving mental illness: stress, coping and adaptation,* New York, 1993, Guilford.

Hoff L: *People in crisis: understanding and helping,* San Francisco, 1995, Jossey-Bass.

Lamb H: A century and a half of psychiatric rehabilitation in the United States, *Hosp Comm Psychiatry* 45:1015, 1994.

Lefley H: Thinking about recovery: paradigms and pitfalls, *Innovations Research* 3:21, 1994.

Mann N et al: Psychosocial rehabilitation in schizophrenia beginnings in acute hospitalization, *Arch Psychiatr Nurs* 7:154, 1993.

Mrazek P, Haggerty R: *Reducing risks for mental disorders,* Washington DC, 1994, National Academy Press.

Murray J: *Prevention of anxiety and depression in vulnerable groups,* London, 1995, Gaskell.

Palmer-Erbs V: Psychiatric rehabilitation: a breath of fresh air in a turbulent health-care environment, *J Psychosoc Nurs* 34:16, 1996.

Rankin S, Stallings K: *Patient education: issues, principles, practices,* Philadelphia, 1996, Lippincott.

Salzer M: Consumer empowerment in mental health organizations: concept, benefits and impediments, *Admin Policy Mental Health* 24:425, 1997.

Starkey D et al: Inpatient psychiatric rehabilitation in a state hospital setting, *J Psychosoc Nurs* 35:10, 1997.

Stuart G, Laraia M: *Principles and practice of psychiatric nursing,* ed 6, St Louis, 1998, Mosby.

Sullivan W: A long and winding road: the process of recovery from mental illness, *Innovations Research* 3:19, 1994.

Tudor K: *Mental health promotion,* London, 1996, Routledge.

Weaver JD: *Disasters: mental health interventions,* Sarasota, Fla, 1995, Professional Resource Press.

Zealberg J, Santos A, Puckett J: *Comprehensive emergency mental health care,* Dunmore, Pa, 1996, Norton.

APPLYING PRINCIPLES IN NURSING PRACTICE

Anxiety Responses and Anxiety Disorders

9

Continuum of Anxiety Responses

Anxiety is a diffuse, vague apprehension associated with feelings of uncertainty and helplessness. This emotion has no specific object. It is subjectively experienced and communicated interpersonally. It is different from fear, which is the intellectual appraisal of danger. Anxiety is the emotional response to that appraisal. The capacity to be anxious is necessary for survival, but severe levels of anxiety are incompatible with life (Fig. 9-1). Anxiety disorders are the most common psychiatric problems in the United States (Box 9-1).

The levels of anxiety follow:

1. *Mild anxiety* is associated with the tension of daily living and makes a person alert and increases the person's perceptual field. This anxiety can motivate learning and produce growth and creativity.

2. *Moderate anxiety* allows a person to focus on immediate concerns and blocks out the periphery. It narrows the person's perceptual field. The person thus experiences selective inattention but can focus on more areas if directed to so do.

3. *Severe anxiety* greatly reduces a person's perceptual field. The person tends to focus on a specific detail and not think about anything else. All behavior is aimed at obtaining relief. The person needs much direction to focus on any other area.

4. *Panic level of anxiety* is associated with awe, dread, and terror. Details are blown out of proportion. Because of

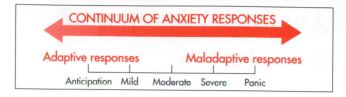

Figure 9-1
Continuum of anxiety responses.

Box 9-1   Prevalence of Anxiety Disorders

- More than 23 million people in the United States are affected by these debilitating illnesses each year, approximately one of every four individuals.
- Anxiety disorders cost the United States $46.6 billion in 1990 in direct and indirect costs, almost one third of the total U.S. mental health bill of $148 billion.
- People with panic disorder spend heavily on health services. One survey found that a patient with panic attacks made an average of 37 medical visits a year, compared with five in the general population.
- Less than 25% of people with panic disorders seek help, mainly because they do not realize their physical symptoms (e.g., heart palpitations, chest pains, shortness of breath) are caused by a psychiatric problem.

---

experiencing a loss of control, the person is unable to do things even with direction. Panic involves the disorganization of the personality and results in increased motor activity, decreased ability to relate to others, distorted perceptions, and loss of rational thought. This level of anxiety is incompatible with life, and if it continues for a long period, exhaustion and death will result.

Assessment

Behaviors

Anxiety can be expressed directly through physiological and behavioral changes and indirectly through the formation of symptoms or coping mechanisms in an attempt to defend against anxiety. The intensity of the behaviors will increase as the level of anxiety increases. Tables 9-1 and 9-2 present the physiological, behavioral, cognitive, and affective responses to anxiety.

Table 9-1   Physiological responses to anxiety

Body System	Responses
Cardiovascular	Palpitations
	Heart "racing"
	Increased blood pressure
	Faintness*
	Actual fainting*
	Decreased blood pressure*
	Decreased pulse rate*
Respiratory	Rapid breathing
	Shortness of breath
	Pressure on chest
	Shallow breathing
	Lump in throat
	Choking sensation
	Gasping
Neuromuscular	Increased reflexes
	Startle reaction
	Eyelid twitching
	Insomnia
	Tremors
	Figidity
	Ridgeting, pacing
	Strained face
	Generalized weakness
	Wobbly legs
	Clumsy movement
Gastrointestinal	Loss of appetite
	Revulsion toward food
	Abdominal discomfort
	Abdominal pain*
	Nausea*
	Heartburn*
	Diarrhea*

*Parasympathetic response.   *Continued*

Table 9-1 Physiological responses to anxiety—cont'd

Body System	Responses
Gastrointestinal	Loss of appetite
	Revulsion toward food
	Abdominal discomfort
	Abdominal pain*
	Nausea*
	Heartburn*
	Diarrhea*
Urinary tract	Pressure to urinate*
	Frequent urination*
Skin	Face flushed
	Localized sweating (palms)
	Itching
	Hot and cold spells
	Face pale
	Generalized sweating

*Parasympathetic response.

Table 9-2 Behavioral, cognitive, and affective responses to anxiety

System	Responses
Behavioral	Restlessness
	Physical tension
	Tremors
	Startle reaction
	Rapid speech
	Lack of coordination
	Accident proneness
	Interpersonal withdrawal
	Inhibition
	Flight
	Avoidance
	Hyperventilation
	Hypervigilance
Cognitive	Impaired attention
	Poor concentration
	Forgetfulness
	Errors in judgment

Table 9-2   Behavioral, cognitive, and affective responses
to anxiety—cont'd

System	Responses
Cognitive—cont'd	Preoccupation
	Blocking of thoughts
	Decreased perceptual field
	Reduced creativity
	Diminished productivity
	Confusion
	Hypervigilence
	Self-consciousness
	Loss of objectivity
	Fear of losing control
	Frightening visual images
	Fear of injury or death
	Flashbacks
	Nightmares
Affective	Edginess
	Impatience
	Uneasiness
	Tension
	Nervousness
	Fearfulness
	Alarm
	Terror
	Jitteriness
	Jumpiness
	Numbness
	Guilt
	Shame

Predisposing Factors

Various theories have been developed to explain the origins of
anxiety:

1. In the *psychoanalytical* view, anxiety is the emotional
   conflict that takes place between two elements of the
   personality: the id and the superego. The id represents
   instinctual drives and primitive impulses, whereas the
   superego reflects conscience and culturally acquired restric-

tions. The ego, or I, serves to mediate the demands of these two opposing elements, and anxiety functions to warn the ego that it is in danger of being overtaken.

2. In the *interpersonal* view, anxiety arises from the fear of interpersonal disapproval and rejection. It is also related to developmental traumas, such as separations and losses, that lead to specific vulnerabilities. People with low self-esteem are particularly vulnerable to the development of high anxiety.

3. In the *behavioral* view, anxiety is a product of frustration, which is anything that interferes with a person's ability to attain a desired goal. Other behaviorists regard anxiety as a learned drive based on an innate desire to avoid pain. Learning theorists believe that individuals who have been exposed in early life to intense fears are more likely to be predisposed to anxiety in later life. Conflict theorists view anxiety as the clashing of two opposing interests. They believe a reciprocal relationship exists between conflict and anxiety: conflict produces anxiety, and anxiety produces feelings of helplessness, which in turn increase the perceived conflict.

4. *Family studies* show that anxiety disorders typically occur within families. Also, anxiety disorders overlap, as do anxiety disorders and depression.

5. *Biological studies* show that the brain contains specific receptors for benzodiazepines, drugs that enhance the inhibitory neuroregulator gamma-aminobutyric acid (GABA), which plays a major role in biological mechanisms relating to anxiety. In addition, a person's general health and a family history of anxiety have a marked effect on predisposition to anxiety. Anxiety may accompany physical disorders and further reduce a person's capacity to cope with stressors.

Precipitating Stressors

Precipitating stressors may be derived from internal or external sources. They can be grouped into the following two categories:

1. *Threats to physical integrity* include impending physiological disability or decreased capacity to perform the activities of daily living.

2. *Threats to self-system* suggest harm to the person's identity, self-esteem, and integrated social functioning.

Appraisal of Stressor

The understanding of anxiety requires integration of many factors, including knowledge from psychoanalytical, interpersonal, behavioral, genetic, and biological perspectives. Appraisal encourages the assessment of patient behaviors and perceptions in developing appropriate nursing interventions. It also suggests a variety of causative factors and stresses the interrelationship among them in explaining the present behavior. Thus a true understanding of anxiety is holistic in nature.

Coping Resources

The individual can cope with stress and anxiety by mobilizing coping resources in the environment. Such coping resources as economic assets, problem-solving abilities, social supports, and cultural beliefs can help the person integrate stressful experiences and adopt successful coping strategies.

Coping Mechanisms

When experiencing anxiety, the individual uses various coping mechanisms to try to allay it, and the inability to cope with anxiety constructively is a primary cause of pathological behavior. The pattern the person typically uses to cope with mild anxiety tends to remain dominant when anxiety becomes more intense. Mild levels of anxiety are often handled without conscious thought. Moderate and severe levels of anxiety elicit the following two types of coping mechanisms:

1. *Task-oriented reactions* are conscious, action-oriented attempts to meet realistically the demands of the stress situation.
- *Attack behavior* is used to remove or overcome an obstacle to satisfy a need.
- *Withdrawal behavior* is used to remove the self either physically or psychologically from the source of the threat.
- *Compromise behavior* is used to change the person's usual way of operating, substitute goals, or sacrifice aspects of personal needs.
2. *Ego defense mechanisms* help to cope with mild and moderate anxiety. Because they operate on a relatively unconscious level and involve a degree of self-deception and reality distortion, however, they can be maladaptive responses to stress. Table 9-3 summarizes some of the most common ego defense mechanisms.

Text continued on p. 172

Table 9-3 Ego defense mechanisms

Defense Mechanism	Definition	Example
Compensation	Process by which a person makes up for a self-image deficiency by strongly emphasizing some other feature the person regards as an asset	Mr. L, a 42-year-old businessman, perceives his small physical stature negatively. He tries to overcome this by being aggressive, forceful, and controlling in his business dealings.
Denial	Avoidance of disagreeable realities by ignoring or refusing to recognize them; probably simplest and most primitive of all defense mechanisms	Mrs. P has just been told that her breast biopsy indicates a malignancy. When her husband visits her that evening, she says that no one has discussed the laboratory results with her.
Displacement	Shift of emotion from a person or object toward which it was originally directed to another usually neutral or less dangerous person or object	Four-year-old Timmy is angry because he has just been punished by his mother for drawing on his bedroom walls. He begins to play "war" with his toy soldiers and has them fight with each other.
Dissociation	Separation of any group of mental or behavioral processes from the rest of consciousness or identity	A man brought to the emergency room by the police is unable to explain who he is and where he lives or works.

Identification	Process by which a person tries to become like someone the person admires by taking on the other's thoughts, mannerisms, or tastes	Sally, 15 years old, has her hair styled similarly to her young English teacher, whom she admires.
Intellectualization	Excessive reasoning or logic used to avoid experiencing disturbing feelings	A woman avoids dealing with her anxiety in shopping malls by explaining that she is saving time and money by not going into them.
Introjection	Intense type of identification in which a person incorporates qualities or values of another person or group into own ego structure; one of the earliest mechanisms of children; important in formation of conscience	Eight-year-old Jimmy tells his 3-year-old sister, "Don't scribble in your book of nursery rhymes. Just look at the pretty pictures."
Isolation	Splitting off of emotional components of a thought, which may be temporary or long term	A second-year medical student dissects a cadaver for her anatomy course without being disturbed by thoughts of death.
Projection	Attributing own thoughts or impulses, particularly intolerable wishes, emotional feelings, or motivations, to another person	A young woman who denies she has sexual feelings about a co-worker accuses him of trying to seduce her.

Continued

Table 9-3 Ego defense mechanisms—cont'd

Defense Mechanism	Definition	Example
Rationalization	Offering a socially acceptable or apparently logical explanation to justify unacceptable impulses, feelings, behaviors, and motives	John fails an examination and complains that the lectures were not well organized or clearly presented.
Reaction formation	Development of conscious attitudes and behavior patterns that are opposite to what a person really feels or would like to do	A married woman who feels attracted to one of her husband's friends treats him rudely.
Regression	Retreat to behavior charactistic of an earlier level of development when confronted by stress	Four-year-old Nicole, who has been toilet-trained for over a year, begins to wet her pants again when her new baby brother is brought home from the hospital.
Repression	Involuntary exclusion of a painful or conflict-ual thought, impulse, or memory from awareness; the primary ego defense, which other mechanisms tend to reinforce	Mr. T does not recall hitting his wife when she was pregnant.
Splitting	Viewing people and situations as either all good or all bad; failure to integrate the positive and negative qualities of the self	A friend tells you that you are the most wonderful person in the world one day, then how much she hates you the next day.

Sublimation	Acceptance of a socially approved substitute goal for a drive whose normal channel of expression is blocked	Ed has an impulsive or physically aggressive nature. He tries out for the football team and becomes a star tackle.
Suppression	Process often listed as a defense mechanism, but really a conscious analogue of repression; intentional exclusion of material from consciousness; at times, may lead to subsequent repression	A young man at work finds he is thinking so much about his date that evening that it is interfering with his work. He decides to put it out of his mind until he leaves the office for the day.
Undoing	Act or communication that partially negates a previous one; primitive defense mechanism	Larry makes a passionate declaration of love to Sue on a date. On their next meeting he treats her formally and distantly.

Nursing Diagnosis

The formulation of a nursing diagnosis requires that the nurse determine the quality (appropriateness) of the patient's response, the quantity (level) of the patient's anxiety, and the adaptive or maladaptive nature of the coping mechanism used.

The box below presents the primary and related NANDA nursing diagnoses for anxiety responses. A complete nursing assessment would include all maladaptive responses of the patient. Many additional nursing problems would be identified in the way that the patient's anxiety reciprocally influenced other areas of life.

NANDA Nursing Diagnoses Related to Anxiety Responses

Adjustment, impaired
*Anxiety
Breathing pattern, ineffective
Communication, impaired verbal
Community coping, ineffective
Confusion, acute
*Coping, ineffective individual
Diarrhea
Energy field disturbance
*Fear
Health maintenance, altered
Injury, risk for
Memory, impaired
Nutrition, altered
Posttrauma response
Powerlessness
Self-esteem disturbance
Sensory/perceptual alterations (specify)
Sleep pattern disturbance
Social interaction, impaired
Thought processes, altered
Urinary elimination, altered

From North American Nursing Diagnosis Association: *NANDA nursing diagnoses: definitions and classification 1997-1998,* Philadelphia, 1998, The Association.
*Primary nursing diagnosis for anxiety.

Related Medical Diagnoses

Many patients experiencing transient or less severe anxiety have no medically diagnosed health problem. However, patients with more severe levels of anxiety most often have neurotic disorders that fall into the category of anxiety disorders in DSM-IV. The box on pp. 174-176 describes these disorders.

Outcome Identification

The expected outcome for patients with maladaptive anxiety responses follows:

The patient will demonstrate adaptive ways of coping with stress.

Planning

Patients need to develop the capacity to tolerate mild anxiety and use it consciously and constructively. In this way the self will become stronger and more integrated. A Patient Education Plan for teaching the relaxation response is presented on pp. 179 and 180.

Implementation

Intervening in Severe and Panic Levels of Anxiety

The highest priority nursing goals should address lowering the patient's severe or panic levels of anxiety, and related nursing interventions should be supportive and protective. A Nursing Treatment Plan Summary related to severe and panic levels of anxiety is presented on pp. 181-183.

Intervening in a Moderate Level of Anxiety

When a patient's anxiety is reduced to the mild or moderate level, the nurse may implement insight-oriented or reeducative nursing interventions. These interventions involve the patient in a problem-solving process and are described in the Nursing Treatment Plan Summary for moderate anxiety on pp. 184-186.

Evaluation

1. Have threats to the patient's physical integrity or self-system been reduced in nature, number, origin, or timing?

Text continued on p. 178

DSM-IV Medical Diagnoses Related to Anxiety Responses

DSM-IV Diagnosis

Panic disorder without agoraphobia

Panic disorder with agoraphobia

Agoraphobia without history of panic disorder

Essential Features

Recurrent unexpected panic attacks (Box 9-2) and at least one of the attacks has been followed by a month (or more) of (1) persistent concern about having additional attacks, (2) worry about the implications of the attack or its consequences, or (3) a significant change in behavior related to the attacks. Also the absence of agoraphobia.

Meets the above criteria. In addition, the presence of agoraphobia, which is anxiety about being in places or situations from which escape might be difficult (or embarrassing) or in which help may not be available in the event of having an unexpected or situationally predisposed panic attack. Agoraphobic fears typically involve characteristic clusters of situations that include being outside the home alone; being in a crowd or standing in a line; being on a bridge; and traveling in a bus, train, or car. Agoraphobic situations are avoided, or are endured with marked distress or with anxiety about having a panic attack, or require the presence of a companion.

Presence of agoraphobia and has never met criteria for panic disorder.

Specific phobia	Marked and persistent fear that is excessive or unreasonable, cued by the presence or anticipation of a specific object or situation (e.g., flying, heights, animals, receiving an injection, seeing blood). Exposure to the phobic stimulus almost invariably provokes an immediate anxiety response. The person recognizes the fear is excessive, and the distress or avoidance interferes with the person's normal routines.
Social phobia	Marked and persistent fear of one or more social or performance situations in which the person is exposed to unfamiliar people or to possible scrutiny by others. The individual fears that he or she will act in a way (or show anxiety symptoms) that will be humiliating or embarrassing. Exposure to the feared situation almost invariably provokes anxiety. The person recognizes the fear is excessive, and the distress or avoidance interferes with the person's normal routine.
Obsessive-compulsive disorder	Either obsessions or compulsions (Box 9-3) are recognized as excessive and interfere with the person's normal routine.
Posttraumatic stress disorder	The person has been exposed to a traumatic event in which both the following occurred:

Continued

DSM-IV Medical Diagnoses Related to Anxiety Responses—cont'd

DSM-IV Diagnosis	Essential Features
Posttraumatic stress disorder—cont'd	1. The person experienced, witnessed, or was confronted with an event or events that involved actual or threatened death or serious injury or a threat to the physical integrity of self or others. 2. The person's response involved intense fear, helplessness, or horror. The person reexperiences the traumatic event, avoids stimuli associated with the trauma, and experiences a numbing of general responsiveness.
Acute stress disorder	Meets the above criteria for exposure to a traumatic event, and the person experiences three of the following symptoms: sense of detachment, reduced awareness of surroundings, derealization, depersonalization, and dissociated amnesia.
Generalized anxiety disorder	Excessive anxiety and worry, occurring more days than not for at least 6 months, about a number of events or activities. The person finds it difficult to control the worry and experiences at least three of the following six symptoms: restlessness or feeling keyed up or on edge, being easily fatigued, difficulty concentrating or mind going blank, irritability, muscle tension, and sleep disturbance.

Modified from American Psychiatric Association: *Diagnostic and statistical manual of mental disorders*, ed 4 (DSM-IV), Washington, DC, 1994, The Association.

Box 9-2   Criteria For Panic Attacks

A panic attack is a discrete period of intense fear or discomfort in which at least four of the following symptoms develop abruptly and reach a peak within 10 minutes:

1. Palpitations, pounding heart, or accelerated heart rate
2. Sweating
3. Trembling or shaking
4. Sensations of shortness of breath or smothering
5. Feeling of choking
6. Chest pain or discomfort
7. Nausea or abdominal distress
8. Feeling dizzy, unsteady, lightheaded, or faint
9. Derealization (feelings of unreality) or depersonalization (being detached from self)
10. Fear of losing control or going crazy
11. Fear of dying
12. Paresthesias (numbness or tingling sensations)
13. Chills or hot flushes

Box 9-3   Criteria For Obsessions and Compulsions

Obsessions

1. Recurrent and persistent thoughts, impulses, or images are experienced at some time during the disturbance as intrusive and inappropriate and cause marked anxiety or distress.
2. The thoughts, impulses, or images are not simply excessive worries about real-life problems.
3. The person attempts to ignore or suppress such thoughts or impulses or to neutralize them with some other thought or action.
4. The person recognizes that the obsessional thoughts, impulses, or images are a product of own mind.

Continued

Box 9-3 Criteria For Obsessions and Compulsions—cont'd

Compulsions

1. The person feels driven to perform repetitive behaviors (e.g., handwashing, ordering, checking) or mental acts (e.g., praying, counting, repeating words silently) in response to an obsession or according to rigidly applied rules.
2. The behaviors or mental acts are aimed at preventing or reducing distress or preventing some dreaded event or situation; however, these behaviors or mental acts are not connected realistically with what they are designed to neutralize or prevent, or they are clearly excessive.

2. Do the patient's behaviors reflect a mild or less severe level of anxiety?
3. Have the patient's coping resources been adequately assessed and mobilized?
4. Does the patient recognize own anxiety and have insight into feelings?
5. Is the patient using adaptive coping responses?
6. Has the patient learned new adaptive strategies to reduce anxiety?
7. Is the patient using mild anxiety to promote personal change and growth?

Patient Education Plan
Teaching the Relaxation Response

Content	Instructional activities	Evaluation
Describe characteristics and benefits of relaxation.	Discuss physiological changes associated with relaxation and contrast these with anxiety behaviors.	Patient identifies own responses to anxiety. Patient describes elements of a relaxed state.
Teach deep muscle relaxation through sequence of tension-relaxation exercises.	Engage patient in progressive procedure of tensing and relaxing muscles until whole body is relaxed.	Patient can tense and relax all muscle groups. Patient identifies those muscles that become particularly tense.
Discuss relaxation procedure of meditation and its components.	Describe elements of meditation and assist patient in using this technique.	Patient selects word or scene with pleasant connotations and engages in relaxed meditation.

Continued

Patient Education Plan
Teaching the Relaxation Response—cont'd

Content	Instructional activities	Evaluation
Assist in overcoming anxiety-provoking situations through systematic desensitization.	With patient, construct hierarchy of anxiety-provoking situations or scenes.	Patient identifies and ranks anxiety-provoking situations.
	Through imagination or reality, work through these scenes, using relaxation techniques.	Patient exposes self to these situations while remaining relaxed.
Allow rehearsing and practical use of relaxation in a safe environment.	Have patient role-play stressful situations with you or other patients.	Patient becomes more comfortable with new behavior in a safe and supportive setting.
Encourage patient to use relaxation techniques in life.	Assign use of the relaxation response in everyday experiences as homework.	Patient uses relaxation in real-life situations.
	Support success of patient who uses relaxation in life situation.	Patient is able to regulate anxiety response through use of relaxation techniques.

Nursing Treatment Plan Summary
Severe and Panic Anxiety Responses

Nursing Diagnosis: Severe/panic level of anxiety
Expected Outcome: Patient will reduce anxiety to a moderate or mild level.

Short-term Goals	Interventions	Rationale
Patient will be protected from harm.	Initially accept and support, rather than attack, patient's defenses. Acknowledge reality of the pain associated with patient's present coping mechanisms. Do not focus on the phobia, ritual, or physical complaint itself. Give feedback to patient about behavior, stressors and their appraisal, and coping resources. Reinforce idea that physical health is related to emotional health and that this area will need exploration in the future. In time, begin to place limits on patient's maladaptive behavior in a supportive way.	Severe and panic levels of anxiety can be reduced by initially allowing patient to determine amount of stress that can be handled. If patient is unable to release anxiety, tension may mount to the panic level and patient may lose control. At this time, patient has no alternatives for present coping mechanisms.

Continued

Nursing Treatment Plan Summary
Severe and Panic Anxiety Responses—cont'd

Short-term Goals	Interventions	Rationale
Patient will experience fewer anxiety-provoking situations.	Assume a calm manner with patient. Decrease environmental stimulation. Limit patient's interaction with other patients to minimize contagious aspects of anxiety. Identify and modify anxiety-provoking situations for patient. Administer supportive physical measures, such as warm baths and massages.	Patient's behavior may be modified by altering environment and patient's interaction with it.

Patient will engage in a daily schedule of activities.	Initially share an activity with patient to provide support and reinforce socially productive behavior.	By encouraging outside activities, nurse limits the time patient has available for destructive coping mechanisms while increasing participation in and enjoyment of other aspects of life.
	Provide for physical exercise of some type.	
	Plan a schedule or list of activities that can be carried out daily.	
	Involve family members and other support systems as much as possible.	
Patient will experience relief from the symptoms of severe anxiety.	Administer medications that help reduce patient's discomfort.	Effect of a therapeutic relationship may be enhanced if chemical control of symptoms allows patient to direct attention to underlying conflicts.
	Observe for medication side effects and initiate relevant health teaching.	

Nursing Treatment Plan Summary
Moderate Anxiety Responses

Nursing Diagnosis: Moderate level of anxiety

Expected Outcome: Patient will demonstrate adaptive ways of coping with stress.

Short-term Goals	Interventions	Rationale
Patient will identify and describe feelings of anxiety.	Help patient identify and describe underlying feelings. Link patient's behavior with such feelings. Validate all inferences and assumptions with patient. Use open questions to move from non-threatening topics to issues of conflict. Vary amount of anxiety to enhance patient's motivation. In time, use supportive confrontation judiciously.	To adopt new coping responses, patient first needs to be aware of feelings and to overcome conscious or unconscious denial and resistance.

Patient will identify antecedents of anxiety.	Help patient describe the situations and interactions that immediately precede anxiety.	Once feelings of anxiety are recognized, patient needs to understand their development, including precipitating stressors, appraisal of the stressor, and available resources.
	Review patient's appraisal of the stressor, values being threatened, and way in which the conflict developed.	
	Relate patient's present experiences with relevant ones from the past.	
Patient will describe adaptive and maladaptive coping responses.	Explore how patient reduced anxiety in the past and what types of actions produced relief.	New adaptive coping responses can be learned through analyzing coping mechanisms used in the past, reappraising the stressor, using available resources, and accepting responsibility for change.
	Point out maladaptive and destructive effects of present coping responses.	
	Encourage patient to use adaptive coping responses that were effective in the past.	
	Focus responsibility for change on patient.	
	Actively help patient correlate cause-and-effect relationships while maintaining anxiety within appropriate limits.	
	Assist patient in reappraising value, nature, and meaning of the stressor when appropriate.	

Continued

Nursing Treatment Plan Summary
Moderate Anxiety Responses—cont'd

Short-term Goals	Interventions	Rationale
Patient will implement two adaptive responses for coping with anxiety.	Help patient identify ways to restructure thoughts, modify behavior, use resources, and test new coping responses. Encourage physical activity to discharge energy. Include significant others as resources and social supports in helping patient learn new coping responses. Teach patient relaxation exercises to increase control and self-reliance and reduce stress.	A person can also cope with stress by regulating the attendant emotional distress through use of stress management techniques.

your **INTERNET**
c o n n e c t i o n

NAPD News: National Panic/Anxiety Disorder News
http://www.npadnews.com
Noodles' Panic-Anxiety Page:
The ANXIETY-Panic Internet Resource http://
www.algy.com/anxiety

Suggested readings

Beck CT: A concept analysis of panic, *Arch Psychiatr Nurs* 5:265, 1996.

Benham E: Coping strategies: a psychoeducational approach to post-traumatic symptomatology, *J Psychosoc Nurs* 6:30, 1995.

Brown P, Yantis J: Personal space intrusion and PTSD, *J Psychosoc Nurs* 24:23, 1996.

Bystritsky A et al: A preliminary study of partial hospital management of severe obsessive-compulsive disorder, *Psychiatric Serv* 47:170, 1996.

Freedy J, Hobfoll S: *Traumatic stress: from theory to practice,* New York, 1995, Plenum Press.

Glod C, McEnany: The neurobiology of posttraumatic stress disorder, *J Am Psychiatr Nurs Assoc* 1:196, 1995.

Mavissakalian MR, Prien RF: *Long term treatments of anxiety disorders,* Washington, DC, 1996, American Psychiatric Press.

Menninger WW: Challenges to providing integrated treatment of anxiety disorders, *Bull Menninger Clin* 58:A86, 1995.

Post-traumatic stress disorder. Parts I and II, *Harvard Ment Health Lett* 12:1, 13:1, 1996.

Roth S: The panic-agoraphobic syndrome: a paradigm of the anxiety group of disorders and its implications for psychiatric practice and theory, *Am J Psychiatry* 153:111, 1996.

Smith S, Sherril K, Colenda C: Assessing and treating anxiety in elderly persons, *Psychiatric Serv* 46:36, 1995.

Stuart G, Laraia M: Panic disorder with agoraphobia. In McBride AB, Austin JK: *Psychiatric–mental health nursing: integrating the behavioral and biological sciences,* Philadelphia, 1996, WB Saunders.

Stuart G, Laraia M: *Principles and practice of psychiatric nursing,* ed 6, St Louis, 1998, Mosby.

Symes L: Post traumatic stress disorder: an evolving concept, *Arch Psychiatr Nurs* 4:195, 1995.

Turner D: Panic disorder: a personal and nursing perspective, *J Psychosoc Nurs* 33:5, 1995.

Waddell K, Demi A: Effectiveness of an intensive partial hospitalization program for treatment of anxiety disorders, *Arch Psychiatr Nurs* 7:2, 1993.

Psycho-physiological Responses and Somatoform and Sleep Disorders

10

Continuum of Psychophysiological Responses

The degree of interconnection between mind and body has always been of interest to scientists and philosophers. For a long time in the history of medicine, body and mind were viewed as separate. More recently, renewed attention has been given to the interrelationship between these two separate aspects of human functioning. Much of the research has focused on the stress response and the impact of stress, including the effect of psychological stress on physiological functioning, and vice versa.

One of the prominent investigators of the stress response, Hans Selye, described the general adaptation syndrome, a three-stage process of responding to stress, as follows:

1. *The alarm reaction.* This is the immediate response to a stressor that has not been eliminated locally. Adrenocortical response mechanisms are mobilized, resulting in the behaviors associated with the fight-or-flight response.
2. *Stage of resistance.* In this stage there is some resistance to the stressor. The body adapts at a lower than optimum level of functioning, requiring greater than usual expenditure of energy for survival.
3. *Stage of exhaustion.* The adaptive mechanisms become worn out and fail in this stage. The negative effect of the stressor

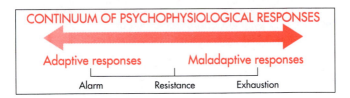

Figure 10-1
Continuum of psychophysiological responses.

> spreads to the entire organism. If the stressor is not removed or counteracted, death will ultimately result.

Fig. 10-1 illustrates the range of possible psychophysiological responses to stress based on Selye's theory.

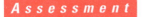

A s s e s s m e n t

Behaviors

Many behaviors are associated with psychophysiological disorders. Careful assessment is needed to define and treat actual organic problems. This type of illness should never be dismissed as "only psychosomatic" or "all in one's head." Serious psychophysiological disorders can be fatal if not treated appropriately.

Physiological

The primary behaviors observed with psychophysiological responses are the physical symptoms. These symptoms lead the person to seek health care. Psychological factors affecting the physical condition may involve any body part. Box 10-1 lists the most common organ systems involved.

Psychological

Some people have physical symptoms without any organic impairment. These *somatoform disorders* include the following:
1. *Somatization disorder,* in which the person has many physical complaints
2. *Conversion disorder,* in which a loss or alteration of physical functioning occurs
3. *Hypochondriasis,* the fear or belief that the person has an illness

Box 10-1   Physical Conditions Affected by Psychological Factors

Cardiovascular

Migraine
Essential hypertension
Angina
Tension headaches

Musculoskeletal

Rheumatoid arthritis
Low back pain (idiopathic)

Gastrointestinal

Anorexia nervosa
Peptic ulcer
Irritable bowel syndrome
Colitis
Obesity

Respiratory

Hyperventilation
Asthma

Skin

Neurodermatitis
Eczema
Psoriasis
Pruritus

Genitourinary

Impotence
Frigidity
Premenstrual syndrome

Endocrinological

Hyperthyroidism
Diabetes

---

4. *Body dysmorphic disorder,* in which a person with a normal appearance is concerned about having a physical defect
5. *Pain disorder,* in which psychological factors play an important role in the onset, severity, or maintenance of the pain

Pain

Pain is increasingly recognized as more than a sensory phenomenon, but as a complex sensory and emotional experience underlying potential disease. Pain is influenced by behavioral, cognitive, motivational, and cultural processes and thus requires sophisticated assessments and multifaceted treatments for its control. By definition, chronic pain consists of pain of at least 6 months' duration. *Somatoform pain disorder* is a preoccupation with pain without physical disease to account for its intensity. It does not follow a neuroanatomical distribution. A close correlation also may exist between stress and conflict and the initiation or exacerbation of the pain.

Sleep

Sleep disturbances are common in the general population and among people with psychiatric disorders. Insomnia is the most prevalent sleep disorder. Up to 30% of the population have insomnia and seek help for it. Other sleep disturbances include excessive daytime sleepiness, difficulty sleeping during desired sleep time, and unusual nocturnal events such as nightmares and sleepwalking. The consequences of sleep disorders, sleep deprivation, and sleepiness include reduced productivity, lowered cognitive performance, increased likelihood of accidents, higher risk of morbidity and mortality, and decreased quality of life. Sleep disorders are more common in elderly persons.

Sleep disorders are classified into the following four major groupings:

1. Disorders of initiating or maintaining sleep, also known as **insomnia.** Anxiety and depression are major causes of insomnia.
2. Disorders of excessive somnolence, also known as **hypersomnia.** This category includes narcolepsy, sleep apnea, and nocturnal movement disorders such as restless legs.
3. Disorders of the sleep-wake schedule, characterized by normal sleep but at the wrong time. These are transient disturbances often associated with jet lag and work shift changes. They are usually self-limited and resolve as the body readjusts to a new sleep-wake schedule.
4. Disorders associated with sleep stages, also known as **parasomnia.** This category includes diverse conditions such as sleepwalking, night terrors, nightmares, and enuresis. These sleep problems are often experienced by children and can have a significant effect on functioning and well-being.

Predisposing Factors

Biopsychosocial factors believed to influence the individual's psychophysiological response to stress include the following:

1. *Biological factors*
   - Emotions have been linked to the arousal of the neuroendocrine system through the release of corticosteroids; the

actions of neurotransmitter systems; and the changes in postsynaptic receptors in response to stress.
- Genetic factors have been shown to influence the prevalence of some psychophysiological disorders.
- Psychoimmunology explores the connection between the mind and the immune system and is discovering biological factors that influence the way the brain protects itself from cells damaged by trauma, disease, or stress.

2. *Psychological factors*
- The type A personality represents the connection of a personality type to a physiological disorder, in this case, heart disease.
- Other investigators have documented a relationship between personality style and physiological disorders such as hypertension and migraine headaches.
- Physical illness may occur with no evidence of organic impairment. In this case, psychological conflicts and anxiety are suspected to predispose a person to respond somatically.

3. *Sociocultural factors*
- The severity of the person's symptoms is influenced by aspects of the social and cultural environment.
- The symptoms shape and structure the person's social world as the illness, by its very presence, initiates a series of changes in the person's environment. The resulting chain of illness-related, interpersonal events then becomes a part of the social course of the person's illness.

Precipitating Stressors

Psychophysiological illnesses result from an attempt to cope with anxiety. Therefore the stressors related to the psychological responses to anxiety discussed in Chapter 9 also apply to the physiological response. The precipitating stressor may be one overwhelming experience or may seem relatively minor. Interpersonal losses are often associated with the development of physical symptoms. Sometimes a psychophysiological illness results from an accumulation of apparently minor stressful events.

Appraisal of Stressor

The complex interaction between mind and body may be most evident in psychophysiological responses to stress. These resulting illnesses reinforce the need for an integrated approach to determining etiology and understanding a person's appraisal of stress and its effects. Social and cultural factors play a particularly important role in the expression of adaptive and maladaptive behaviors and must be prime considerations in planning effective, individualized treatment strategies.

Coping Resources

One of the most important aspects of promoting adaptive psychophysiological responses involves changing health habits. Social support from family, friends, and caregivers is also an important resource.

Coping Mechanisms

The psychophysiological disorders may be viewed as attempts to cope with the anxiety associated with overwhelming stress. Ego defense mechanisms associated with these disorders include the following:

1. Repression of feelings, conflicts, and unacceptable impulses
2. Denial of psychological problems
3. Compensation
4. Regression

Nursing Diagnosis

The nursing diagnosis must reflect the complexity of the biopsychosocial interaction, which is the hallmark of psychophysiological disorders. The individual's effort to cope with stress-related anxiety may result in numerous somatic and emotional disorders. Care must be taken to consider all the possible disruptions when formulating a complete nursing diagnosis.

The box on p. 194 presents the primary and related NANDA nursing diagnoses for maladaptive psychophysiological responses. A complete nursing assessment would include all maladaptive responses of the patient, and many additional nursing diagnoses would be identified.

Related Medical Diagnoses

Medical disorders related to psychophysiological responses are classified under the general headings of somatoform disorders,

NANDA Nursing Diagnoses Related to Maladaptive Psychophysiological Responses

*Adjustment, impaired
 Anxiety
 Body image disturbance
 Coping, ineffective individual
 Denial, ineffective
 Family processes, altered
 Fear
 Gas exchange, impaired
 Health maintenance, altered
 Hopelessness
 Mobility, impaired physical
 Nutrition, altered: less than body requirements
*Pain, chronic
 Powerlessness
 Self-care deficit (specify)
 Self-esteem disturbance
 Skin integrity, impaired
*Sleep pattern disturbance
 Social interaction, impaired
 Social isolation
 Spiritual distress

From North American Nursing Diagnosis Association: *NANDA nursing diagnoses: definitions and classification 1997-1998,* Philadelphia, 1997, The Association.
*Primary nursing diagnosis for maladaptive psychophysiological responses.

sleep disorders, and psychological factors affecting medical condition in DSM-IV. The box on pp. 196-197 describes somatoform and sleep disorders.

Outcome Identification

The expected outcome when working with a patient with maladaptive psychophysiological responses follows:

The patient will express feelings verbally rather than through the development of physical symptoms.

Planning

A Patient Education Plan for teaching adaptive coping strategies is presented on pp. 198 and 199.

Implementation

Intervening in Psychophysiological Illness

The highest priority for nursing intervention is attending to the patient's physiological needs. This assists the patient to meet basic needs for safety and security. It is also valuable for fostering the development of a trusting relationship. Box 10-2 presents sleep hygiene strategies. A Nursing Treatment Plan Summary for patients with maladaptive psychophysiological responses is presented on pp. 201 and 202.

Evaluation

1. Have threats to the patient's physical integrity or self-system been reduced in nature, origin, or timing?
2. Do the patient's behaviors reflect greater self-awareness and acceptance of emotional experiences?
3. Have the patient's coping resources been adequately assessed and mobilized?
4. Does the patient recognize the level of stress, and does the patient have insight into own feelings?
5. Is the patient using adaptive coping responses?
6. Has the patient learned new adaptive strategies to cope effectively with life stressors?
7. Is the patient using greater self-understanding to promote personal change and growth?

DSM-IV Medical Diagnoses Related to Maladaptive Psychophysiological Responses

DSM-IV Diagnosis	Essential Features
Somatization disorder	History of many physical complaints beginning before age 30, occurring over several years, and resulting in treatment being sought or significant impairment in social or occupational functioning. The patient must display at least four pain symptoms, two gastrointestinal symptoms, one sexual symptom, and one symptom suggesting a neurological disorder.
Conversion disorder	One or more symptoms or deficits affecting voluntary motor or sensory function and suggesting a neurological or general medical condition. Psychological factors are judged to be associated with the symptom or deficit because the initiation or exacerbation of the symptom or deficit is preceded by conflicts or other stressors. The symptom or deficit cannot be fully explained by a neurological or general medical condition and is not a culturally sanctioned behavior or experience.
Hypochondriasis	Preoccupation with fears of having, or ideas that one has, a serious disease based on the person's misinterpretation of bodily symptoms. The preoccupation persists for at least 6 months despite appropriate medical evaluation and reassurance. It causes clinically significant distress or impairment in functioning.
Body dysmorphic disorder	Preoccupation with an imagined or exaggerated defect in appearance that causes clinically significant distress or impairment in functioning.

Pain disorder	Pain in one or more anatomical sites is predominant focus of the clinical presentation. It is of sufficient severity to warrant clinical attention and causes clinically significant distress or impairment in functioning. Psychological factors are judged to have an important role in the onset, severity, exacerbation, or maintenance of the pain.
Primary insomnia	Difficulty initiating or maintaining sleep, or nonrestorative sleep, for at least 1 month that causes clinically significant distress or impairment in functioning.
Primary hypersomnia	Excessive sleepiness for at least 1 month, as evidenced by either prolonged sleep episodes or daytime sleep episodes occurring almost daily, that causes clinically significant distress or impairment in functioning.
Narcolepsy	Irresistible attacks of refreshing sleep occurring daily over at least 3 months with cataplexy (brief episodes of sudden bilateral loss of muscle tone) and hallucinations or sleep paralysis at the beginning or end of sleep episodes.
Breathing-related sleep disorder	Sleep disruption leading to excessive sleepiness or insomnia judged to be caused by sleep apnea or central alveolar hypoventilation syndrome.
Circadian rhythm sleep disorder	Persistent or recurrent pattern of sleep disruption leading to excessive sleepiness or insomnia that is caused by a mismatch between the sleep-wake schedule required by a person's environment and the circadian sleep-wake pattern and that causes clinically significant distress or impairment in functioning.
Psychological factors affecting medical condition	Presence of a medical condition in which psychological factors influence its cause, interfere with its treatment, constitute additional health risks for the individual, or elicit stress-related physiological responses that precipitate or exacerbate its symptoms.

Modified from American Psychiatric Association: *Diagnostic and statistical manual of mental disorders*, ed 4 (DSM-IV), Washington, DC, 1994, The Association.

Patient Education Plan
Teaching Adaptive Coping Strategies

Content	Instructional Activities	Evaluation
Define and describe stress.	List feelings that indicate stress. Discuss behaviors associated with elevated stress.	Patient identifies behaviors associated with stressful situations.
Recognize stressful situations.	Ask patient to describe situations experienced as stressful. Role-play the situation (with videotape if possible). Discuss stress-related behaviors observed and feelings experienced.	Patient identifies stressful experiences. Patient describes own behaviors when stressed.
Review common life stressors.	Discuss common elements of stressful experiences.	Patient identifies stressful aspects of life.

Patient identifies and practices adaptive coping mechanisms.

Patient selects an adaptive coping strategy when experiencing stress.

Review the role-played stressful situations.

Discuss alternative ways to cope with the stressors.

Role-play at least one coping mechanism.

Provide feedback about effectiveness of the selected coping mechanism.

Identify adaptive and maladaptive coping mechanisms.

Assign use of adaptive strategy to cope with stress.

Box 10-2   Sleep Hygiene Strategies

- Set a regular bedtime and wake-up time 7 days a week.
- Exercise daily to aid sleep initiation and maintenance; however, vigorous exercise too close to bedtime may make falling asleep difficult.
- Schedule time to wind down and relax before bed.
- Avoid worrying when trying to fall asleep.
- Guard against nighttime interruptions. Earplugs may help with a noisy partner. Heavy window shades help to screen out light. Create a comfortable bed.
- Maintain a cool temperature in the room. A warm bath or warm drink before bed helps some people fall asleep.
- Excessive hunger or fullness may interfere with sleep. Avoid large meals before bed. If hungry, a light carbohydrate snack may be helpful.
- Avoid caffeinated drinks, excessive fluid intake, stimulating drugs, and excessive alcohol in the evening and before bedtime.
- Excessive napping may make it difficult for some people to fall asleep at night.
- Do not eat, read, work, or watch television in bed. The bed and bedroom should be used only for sleep and sex.
- Maintain a reasonable weight. Excessive weight may result in daytime fatigue and sleep apnea.
- Get out of bed and engage in other activities if not able to fall asleep.

Nursing Care Plan Summary
Maladaptive Psychophysiological Responses

Nursing Diagnosis: Impaired adjustment
Expected Outcome: Patient will express feelings verbally rather than through the development of physical symptoms.

Short-term Goals	Interventions	Rationale
Patient will identify areas of stress and conflict and relate feelings, thoughts, and behaviors to them.	Assist patient in identifying stressful situations by reviewing events surrounding the development of physical symptoms. Facilitate the association among thoughts, feelings, and behaviors.	Inability to deal with intrapsychic conflict leads to anxiety and stress, resulting in physiological dysfunction.
Patient will describe present defenses and evaluate whether they are adaptive or maladaptive.	Proceed slowly in analyzing defenses. Explore alternative coping behaviors with patient. Teach patient stress management techniques (e.g., relaxation, imagery).	Defenses should not be attacked; rather, nurse should support positive exploration of patient and suggest alternative responses.

Continued

Nursing Care Plan Summary
Maladaptive Psychophysiological Responses—cont'd

Short-term Goals	Interventions	Rationale
Patient will adopt two new coping mechanisms to deal with stress.	Give patient positive feedback for new adaptive behaviors.	Change requires time and positive reinforcement from others.
	Actively support patient in testing new coping mechanisms.	Family members can be particularly important in promoting adaptive responses.
	Enlist support of family and significant others to reinforce change.	
Patient will display decreased physical symptoms and greater biological integrity.	Encourage physical activity to reduce stress.	Wellness requires a balance between biological and psychosocial needs.
	Counsel patient on diet and nutrition needs.	Interventions focused on patient's physiological needs can help patient restore biological integrity.
	Review patient's sleep habits and promote good sleep hygiene practices.	

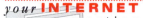

your **INTERNET**
c o n n e c t i o n

Life Sciences Institute of Mind-Body Health
Presents: Self-Regulation of Mind & Body
http://www.cjnetworks.com/~lifesci/
The SLEEP WELL
http://www-leland.stanford.edu/~dement/

Suggested readings

Birch S, Hammerschlag R, Berman B: Acupuncture in the treatment of pain, *J Altern Complement Med* 2:101, 1996.

Blumenthal S, Fine T: Sleep abnormalities associated with mental and addictive disorders: implications for research and clinical practice, *J Pract Psychiatry Behav Health* 3:67, 1996.

Buysse DJ, Perlis ME: The evaluation and treatment of insomnia, *J Pract Psychiatry Behav Health* 3:80, 1996.

Dossey B: Using imagery to help your patient heal, *AJN* 1995:41, 1995.

Dossey BM, Keegan L, Guzzetta CE, Kolkmeier LG: *Holistic nursing: a handbook for practice,* Gaithersburg, Md, 1995, Aspen.

Holmes E et al: Development of a sleep management program for people with severe mental illness, *Psychiatric Rehab J* 19:9;1995.

Keefe FJ, Goli V: A practical guide to behavioral assessment and treatment of chronic pain, *J Pract Psychiatry Behav Health* 5:151, 1996.

Lowery BJ, Houldin AD: From stressor to illness: the psychobiological-biological connection. In McBride AB, Austin JK, editors: *Psychiatric–mental health nursing: integrating the behavioral and biological sciences,* Philadelphia, 1996, WB Saunders.

Mackey R: Discover the healing power of therapeutic touch, *AJN* 1995:27, 1995.

McCain N, Smith J: Stress and coping in the context of psychoneuroimmunology: a holistic framework for nursing practice and research, *Arch Psychiatric Nurs* 8:221, 1994.

Moore DP, Jefferson JW: *Handbook of medical psychiatry,* St Louis, 1996, Mosby.

Oakley LD, Potter C: *Psychiatric primary care,* St Louis, 1997, Mosby.

Selye H: *The stress of life,* New York, 1956, McGraw-Hill.

Stoudemire A: Psychological factors affecting medical conditions, Washington DC, 1995, American Psychiatric Press.

Stuart G, Laraia M: *Principles and practice of psychiatric nursing,* ed 6, St Louis, 1998, Mosby.

Self-Concept Responses and Dissociative Disorders

11

Continuum of Self-Concept Responses

Self-concept is defined as all the notions, beliefs, and convictions that constitute an individual's knowledge of self and that influence relationships with others. Self-concept does not exist at birth; it is learned as a result of a person's unique experiences within the self, with significant others, and with worldly realities. Self-concept consists of the following components:

1. *Body image*—the sum of the individual's conscious and unconscious attitudes toward one's body. It includes present and past perceptions and feelings about size, function, appearance, and potential. Body image is continually modified by new perceptions and experiences.

2. *Self-ideal*—the individual's perception of how he or she should behave based on certain personal standards, aspirations, goals, or values.

3. *Self-esteem*—the individual's judgment of personal worth obtained by analyzing how well one's behavior conforms to self-ideal. High self-esteem is a feeling rooted in unconditional acceptance of self, despite mistakes, defeats, and failures, as an innately worthy and important being.

4. *Role performance*—sets of socially expected behavior patterns associated with an individual's function in various social groups. Ascribed roles are assigned roles over which the person has no choice. Assumed roles are those selected or chosen by the individual.

5. *Personal identity*—the organizing principle of the personality that accounts for the individual's unity, continuity, consistency, and uniqueness. It connotes autonomy and includes perceptions of one's sexuality. Identity formation begins in infancy and proceeds throughout life but is the major task of the adolescent period.

The Healthy Personality

An individual with a healthy personality would experience the following:
1. Positive and accurate body image
2. Realistic self-ideal
3. Positive self-concept
4. High self-esteem
5. Satisfying role performance
6. Clear sense of identity

The self-concept responses along the health-illness continuum range from the most adaptive state of self-actualization to the more maladaptive states of identity diffusion and depersonalization (Fig. 11-1). *Identity diffusion* is an individual's failure to integrate various childhood identifications into a harmonious adult psychosocial personality. *Depersonalization* is a feeling of unreality and alienation from the self. It is associated with the panic level of anxiety and failure in reality test-

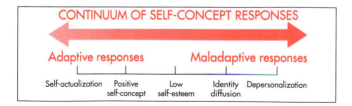

Figure 11-1
Continuum of self-concept responses.

ing. The individual has difficulty distinguishing the self from others, and the person's body has an unreal and strange quality about it.

Assessment

Behaviors

Data collection by the nurse should include both objective and observable behaviors and the patient's subjective and internal world. Boxes 11-1 to 11-3 list behaviors related to low self-esteem, identity diffusion, and depersonalization.

Predisposing Factors

Numerous factors contribute to alterations in an individual's self-concept. These may be divided as follows:

1. *Factors affecting self-esteem* include parental rejection, unrealistic parental expectations, repeated failures, lack of

---

Box 11-1   Behaviors Associated with Low Self-Esteem

Criticism of self and others
Decreased productivity
Destructiveness toward others
Disruptions in relatedness
Exaggerated sense of self-importance
Feelings of inadequacy
Guilt
Irritability or excessive anger
Negative feelings about one's body
Perceived role strain
Pessimistic view of life
Physical complaints
Polarizing view of life
Rejection of personal capabilities
Self-destructiveness
Self-diminution
Social withdrawal
Substance abuse
Withdrawal from reality
Worrying

Box 11-2   Behaviors Associated with Identity Diffusion

Absence of moral code
Contradictory personality traits
Exploitative interpersonal relationships
Feelings of emptiness
Fluctuating feelings about self
Gender confusion
High degree of anxiety
Inability to empathize with others
Lack of authenticity
Problems with intimacy

Box 11-3   Behaviors Associated with Depersonalization

Affective

Feelings of alienation from self
Feelings of insecurity, inferiority, fear, shame
Feelings of unreality
Heightened sense of isolation
Inability to derive pleasure or sense of accomplishment
Lack of sense of inner continuity
Loss of identity

Perceptual

Auditory and visual hallucinations
Confusion about one's sexuality
Difficulty distinguishing self from others
Disturbed body image
Experiencing world as dreamlike

Cognitive

Confusion
Disoriented to time
Distorted thinking
Disturbance of memory
Impaired judgment
Separate personalities within same person

Continued

Box 11-3 Behaviors Associated
with Depersonalization—cont'd

Behavioral

Blunting of affect
Emotional passivity and nonresponsiveness
Incongruent or idiosyncratic communication
Lack of spontaneity and animation
Loss of impulse control
Loss of initiative and decision-making ability
Social withdrawal

personal responsibility, dependency on others, and unrealistic self-ideals.
2. *Factors affecting role performance* are gender role stereotypes, work role demands, and cultural role expectations.
3. *Factors affecting personal identity* include parental distrust, peer pressure, and changes in the social structure.

Precipitating Stressors

Precipitating stressors may be derived from internal or external sources, as follows:
1. *Trauma* such as sexual and psychological abuse or witnessing a life-threatening event
2. *Role strain* associated with expected roles or positions that the person experiences as frustration. The three types of role transitions follow:
   - *Developmental role transitions* are normative changes associated with growth. They include developmental stages in an individual's or family's life and cultural norms, values, and pressures to conform.
   - *Situational role transitions* occur with the addition or subtraction of significant others through birth or death.
   - *Health-illness role transitions* result from moving from a well state to an illness state. Such transitions may be precipitated by the following:
     —Loss of a body part
     —Changes in body size, shape, appearance, or function

—Physical changes associated with normal growth and development

—Medical and nursing procedures

Appraisal of Stressor

Whether the problem in self-concept is precipitated by psychological, sociological, or physiological stressors, the critical element is the patient's perception of the threat.

Coping Resources

All people, no matter how disturbing their behavior, have some areas of personal strength, which might include the following:

- Sports and outdoor activities
- Hobbies and crafts
- Expressive arts
- Health and self-care
- Education or training
- Work, vocation, job, or position
- Special aptitudes
- Intelligence
- Imagination and creativity
- Interpersonal relationships

Coping Mechanisms

Coping mechanisms include short-term or long-term coping defenses and the use of ego defense mechanisms to protect the person from facing painful self-perceptions. *Short-term defenses* include the following:

1. Activities that provide temporary escape from the person's identity crisis (e.g., loud rock concerts, hard physical labor, obsessive television watching)
2. Activities that provide temporary substitute identities (e.g., joining social, religious, or political clubs, groups, movements, or gangs)
3. Activities that serve temporarily to strengthen or heighten a diffuse sense of self (e.g., competitive sports, academic achievement, popularity contests)
4. Activities that represent short-term attempts to make an identity out of the meaninglessness of life itself (e.g., drug abuse)

Long-term defenses include the following:
1. *Identity foreclosure*—the premature adoption of an identity that is desired by significant others without coming to terms with one's own desires, aspirations, or potential
2. *Negative identity*—assumption of an identity that is at odds with accepted values and accepted expectations of society

Ego defense mechanisms include the use of fantasy, dissociation, isolation, projection, displacement, splitting, turning anger against self, and acting out (see Table 9-3).

Nursing Diagnosis

Problems with self-concept are associated with feelings of anxiety, hostility, and guilt. These often create a circular and self-propagating process for the individual that ultimately results in maladaptive coping responses. These responses can be seen in a variety of people experiencing threats to their physical integrity or self-system.

The box on p. 211 presents the primary and related NANDA nursing diagnoses for maladaptive self-concept responses. A complete nursing assessment would include all maladaptive responses of the patient. Many additional nursing problems would be identified in the way that the patient's self-concept reciprocally influenced other areas of life.

Related Medical Diagnoses

Because it pertains to a person's basic personality structure and feelings about the self, the nursing diagnoses related to self-concept can include a variety of medical disorders. A number of specific medical diagnoses have dominant features that relate to one's self-concept. The box on p. 212 identifies and describes these diagnoses.

Outcome Identification

The expected outcome when working with a patient with a maladaptive self-concept response follows:

The patient will obtain the maximum level of self-actualization to realize one's potential.

NANDA Nursing Diagnoses Related to Maladaptive Self-Concept Responses

Adjustment, impaired
Anxiety
*Body image disturbance
Communication, impaired verbal
Coping, ineffective individual
Energy field disturbance
Grieving, dysfunctional
Hopelessness
Loneliness, risk for
*Personal identity disturbance
Powerlessness
*Role performance, altered
Self-care deficit (specify)
*Self-esteem disturbance
Sensory/perceptual alterations (specify)
Sexuality patterns, altered
Social interaction, impaired
Social isolation
Spiritual distress
Spiritual well-being, potential for enhanced
Thought processes, altered
Violence, risk for

From North American Nursing Diagnosis Association: *NANDA nursing diagnoses: definitions and classification 1997-1998,* Philadelphia, 1997, The Association.
*Primary nursing diagnosis for alterations in self-concept.

Planning

A Patient Education Plan for promoting the patient's self-differentiation in the family of origin is presented on p. 213.

Implementation

Intervening in Alterations in Self-Concept

Nursing intervention helps the patient examine his or her cognitive appraisal of the situation and related feelings to help the patient gain

DSM-IV Medical Diagnoses
Related to Maladaptive Self-Concept Responses

DSM-IV Diagnosis	Essential Features
Identity problem	Uncertainty about multiple issues relating to identity, such as long-term goals, career choice, friendship patterns, sexual orientation and behavior, moral values, and group loyalties.
Dissociative amnesia	Predominant disturbance is one or more episodes of inability to recall important personal information, usually of a traumatic or stressful nature, that is too extensive to be explained by ordinary forgetfulness.
Dissociative fugue	Predominant disturbance is sudden, unexpected travel away from home or one's customary place of work, with inability to recall one's past. Confusion about personal identity or assumption of a new identity.
Dissociative identity disorder (multiple personality disorder)	Presence of two or more distinct identities or personality states (each with its own relatively enduring pattern of perceiving, relating to, and thinking about the environment and self). At least two of these identities or personality states recurrently take control of the person's behavior. Inability to recall important personal information that is too extensive to be explained by ordinary forgetfulness.
Depersonalization disorder	Persistent or recurrent experiences of feeling detached from, and as if one is an outside observer of, one's mental processes or body (e.g., feeling as if one is in a dream). During the depersonalization experience, reality testing remains intact. The depersonalization causes clinically significant distress or impairment in functioning.

Modified from American Psychiatric Association: *Diagnostic and statistical manual of mental disorders, ed 4*, (DSM-IV), Washington, DC, 1994, The Association.

Patient Education Plan
Improving Family Relationships

Content	Instructional Activities	Evaluation
Define concept of self-differentiation in a person's family of origin.	Discuss differences between high and low levels of self-differentiation. Ask patient to identify level of functioning among family members.	Patient identifies own functioning level in family of origin.
Describe characteristics of emotional fusion, emotional cutoff, and triangulation.	Analyze types and patterns of family relationships. Use paper and pencil to diagram family patterns.	Patient describes interactional patterns in own family. Patient identifies own roles and behavior.
Discuss role of symptom formation and symptom bearer in a family.	Sensitize patient to family dynamics and manifestations of stress. Encourage family communication. Use a blackboard to map out a family genogram.	Patient recognizes family's contribution to stress of individual members. Patient contacts family members. Patient obtains factual information about family.
Describe a family genogram and show how it is constructed.	Assign family genogram.	Patient constructs family genogram.
Analyze need for objectivity and responsibility for changing own behavior and not that of others.	Role-play interactions with various family members. Encourage testing out new ways of interacting with family members.	Patient demonstrates higher level of differentiation in family of origin.

insight and then take action to bring about behavioral change. This problem-solving approach requires progressive levels of intervention, as follows:

1. Expanded self-awareness
2. Self-exploration
3. Self-evaluation
4. Realistic planning
5. Commitment to action

Tables 11-1 through 11-5 describe specific principles, rationales, and nursing interventions for each progressive level in the sequence. A Nursing Treatment Plan Summary for maladaptive self-concept responses is presented on pp. 224 and 225.

Evaluation

1. Have threats to the patient's physical integrity or self-system been reduced in nature, number, origin, or timing?
2. Do the patient's behaviors reflect greater self-acceptance, self-worth, and self-approval?
3. Have the patient's coping resources been adequately assessed and mobilized?
4. Has the patient expanded self-awareness and engaged in self-exploration and self-evaluation?
5. Is the patient using adaptive coping responses?
6. Has the patient learned new adaptive strategies to enhance the level of self-actualization?
7. Is the patient using greater self-understanding to promote personal change and growth?

Table 11-1   Nursing interventions for alterations in self-concept at level 1

Principle	Rationale	Nursing Interventions
Goal: To Expand Patient's Self-Awareness		
Establish an open, trusting relationship.	Reduce threat that nurse poses to patient; help patient to broaden and accept all aspects of personality.	Offer unconditional acceptance. Listen to patient. Encourage discussion of patient's thoughts and feelings. Respond nonjudgmentally. Convey that patient is a valued person who is responsible for and able to help self.
Work with whatever ego strength patient possesses.	Some degree of ego strength, such as capacity for reality testing, self-control, or a degree of ego integration, is needed as a foundation for later nursing care.	Identify patient's ego strength. Use guidelines for patient with limited ego resources: 1. Begin by confirming patient's identity. 2. Provide support measures to reduce panic level of anxiety. 3. Approach patient in nondemanding way. 4. Accept and attempt to clarify any verbal or nonverbal communication. 5. Prevent patient from isolating self. 6. Establish simple routine for patient. 7. Set limits on inappropriate behavior. 8. Orient patient to reality.

Continued

Table 11-1   Nursing interventions for alterations in self-concept at level 1—cont'd

Principle	Rationale	Nursing Interventions
Goal: To Expand Patient's Self-Awareness—cont'd		
		9. Reinforce appropriate behavior.
		10. Gradually increase activities and tasks that provide positive experiences.
		11. Assist in personal hygiene and grooming.
		12. Encourage patient in self-care.
Maximize patient's participation in therapeutic relationship.	Mutuality is necessary for patient to assume ultimate responsiblity for own behavior and maladaptive coping responses.	Gradually increase patient's participation in care decisions.
		Convey that patient is a responsible individual.

Table 11-2   Nursing interventions for alterations in self-concept at level 2

Principle	Rationale	Nursing Interventions
Goal: To Expand Patient's Self-Exploration		
Assist patient to accept own feelings and thoughts.	By showing interest in and accepting patient's feelings and thoughts, nurse helps patient to do the same.	Attend to and encourage patient's expression of emotions, beliefs, behavior, and thoughts—verbally, nonverbally, symbolically, or directly.
		Use therapeutic communication skills and empathic responses.
		Note patient's use of logical and illogical thinking and reported and observed emotional responses.
Help patient clarify concept of self and relationship to others through self-disclosure.	Self-disclosure and understanding self-perceptions are prerequisites to bringing about future change; this alone may reduce anxiety.	Elicit patient's perception of self-strengths and weaknesses.
		Assist patient to describe self-ideal.
		Identify patient's self-criticisms.
		Help patient to describe beliefs on how he or she relates to other people and events.
Be aware of and have control of own feelings.	Self-awareness allows nurse to model authentic behavior and limits potential negative effects of countertransference in relationship.	Be open to own feelings.
		Accept both positive and negative feelings.
		Practice therapeutic use of self:
		1. Share own feelings with patient.
		2. Verbalize how another might have felt.
		3. Mirror own perception of patient's feelings.

Continued

Table 11-2 Nursing interventions for alterations in self-concept at level 2—cont'd

Principle	Rationale	Nursing Interventions
Goal: To Expand Patient's Self-Exploration—cont'd		
Respond empathically, not sympathetically, emphasizing that power to change lies with patient.	Sympathy can reinforce patient's self-pity; rather, nurse should communicate that patient's life situation is subject to self-control.	Use empathic responses and monitor self for feelings of sympathy or pity.
		Reaffirm that patient is not helpless or powerless in face of problems.
		Convey verbally and behaviorally that patient is responsible for own behavior, including choice of maladaptive or adaptive coping responses.
		Discuss scope of patient's choices, areas of ego strength, and available coping resources.
		Use support systems of family and groups to facilitate patient's self-exploration.
		Assist patient in recognizing nature of conflict and maladaptive coping responses.

Table 11-3   Nursing interventions for alterations in self concept at level 3

Principle	Rationale	Nursing Interventions
Goal: To Expand Patient's Self-Evaluation		
Help patient define the problem clearly.	Only after problem is accurately defined can alternative choices be proposed.	Identify relevant stressors and patient's appraisal of them.
		Clarify that patient's beliefs influence both feelings and behaviors.
		Mutually identify faulty beliefs, misperceptions, distortions, illusions, and unrealistic goals.
		Mutually identify areas of strength.
		Place concepts of success and failure in proper perspective.
		Explore patient's use of coping resources.

Continued

Table 11-3   Nursing interventions for alterations in self concept at level 3—cont'd

Principle	Rationale	Nursing Interventions
Goal: To Expand Patient's Self-Evaluation—cont'd		
Explore patient's adaptive and maladaptive coping responses to the problem.	It is necessary to examine patient's coping choices and evaluate both positive and negative consequences.	Describe to patient how all coping responses are freely chosen and have both positive and negative consequences.
		Contrast adaptive and maladaptive responses.
		Mutually identify disadvantages of patient's maladaptive coping responses.
		Mutually identify advantages, or "payoffs," of patient's maladaptive coping responses.
		Discuss how these payoffs have perpetuated the maladaptive response.
		Use variety of therapeutic skills, such as:
		1. Facilitative communication
		2. Supportive confrontation
		3. Role clarification
		4. Transference and countertransference reaction in the one-to-one relationship
		5. Psychodrama

Table 11-4   Nursing interventions for alterations in self concept at level 4

Principle	Rationale	Nursing Interventions
Goal: To Assist Patient in Formulating a Realistic Plan of Action		
Help patient identify alternative solutions.	Only when all possible alternatives have been evaluated can change be effected.	Help patient understand that only he or she can change self, not others.
		If patient holds inconsistent perceptions, help patient see how to change the following:
		1. Beliefs or ideals to bring them closer to reality
		2. Environment to make it consistent with patient's beliefs
		If self-concept is not consistent with behavior, help patient see how to change the following:
		1. Behavior to conform to self-concept
		2. Beliefs underlying self-concept to include behavior
		3. Self-ideal
		Mutually review how patient may better use coping resources.

Continued

Table 11-4   Nursing interventions for alterations in self concept at level 4—cont'd

Principle	Rationale	Nursing Interventions
Goal: To Assist Patient in Formulating a Realistic Plan of Action—cont'd		
Help patient conceptualize own realistic goals.	Goal setting must include a clear definition of the expected change.	Encourage patient to formulate own (not nurse's) goals.
		Mutually discuss emotional, practical, and reality-based consequences of each goal.
		Help patient clearly define the concrete change to be made.
		Encourage patient to enter new experiences for their growth potential.
		Use role rehearsal, role modeling, role playing, and visualization when appropriate.

Table 11-5   Nursing interventions for alterations in self concept at level 5

Principle	Rationale	Nursing Interventions
Goal: To Assist Patient to Become Committed to Decision and Achieve Own Goals		
Help patient take necessary action to change maladaptive coping responses and maintain adaptive ones.	Ultimate objective in promoting insights is to have patient replace maladaptive coping responses with more adaptive ones.	Provide opportunity for patient to experience success. Reinforce strengths, skills, and healthy aspects of patient's personality. Assist patient in gaining assistance (vocational, financial, socal services) Use groups to enhance patient's self-esteem. Promote patient's self-differentiation in family of origin. Allow patient sufficient time to change. Provide appropriate amount of support and positive reinforcement to help patient maintain progress.

Nursing Treatment Plan Summary
Maladaptive Self-Concept Responses

Nursing Diagnosis: Self-esteem disturbance
Expected Outcome: Patient will obtain the maximum level of self-actualization to realize one's potential.

Short-Term Goals	Interventions	Rationale
Patient will establish a therapeutic relationship with nurse.	Confirm patient's identity.	Mutuality is necessary for patient to assume responsibility for behavior.
	Provide supportive measures to decrease panic level of anxiety.	Some degree of ego integrity is needed for later interventions.
	Set limits on inappropriate behavior.	
	Work with whatever ego strengths patient possesses.	
	Reinforce adaptive behavior.	
Patient will express feelings, behaviors, and thoughts related to present stressful situations.	Assist patient to express and describe feelings and thoughts.	Self-disclosure and understanding are necessary to bring about change.
	Help patient in identifying strengths and weaknesses, self-ideal, and self-criticisms.	Use of sympathy is not therapeutic because it can reinforce patient's self-pity; rather, nurse should communicate that patient is in control.
	Respond empathically, emphasizing that the power to change lies within patient.	

Patient will evaluate the positive and negative consequences of self-concept responses.	Identify relevant stressors and patient's appraisal of them.	Only after the problem is defined can alternative choices be examined; then the positive and negative consequences of current patterns must be evaluated.
	Clarify faulty beliefs and cognitive distortions.	
	Evaluate advantages and disadvantages of current coping responses.	
Patient will identify one new goal and two adaptive coping responses.	Encourage patient to formulate a new goal.	Only after alternatives have been explored can change be effected.
	Help patient clearly define the change to be made.	Goal setting specifies nature of the change and suggests possible new behavioral strategies.
	Use role rehearsal, role modeling, and visualization to practice the new behavior.	
Patient will implement the new adaptive self-concept responses.	Provide opportunity for patient to experience success.	Ultimate goal in promoting patient's insight is to have patient replace the maladaptive coping responses with more adaptive ones.
	Reinforce strengths, skills, and adaptive coping responses.	
	Allow patient sufficient time to change.	
	Promote group and family involvement.	
	Provide appropriate amount of support and positive reinforcement for patient to maintain progress and growth.	

your **INTERNET**
c o n n e c t i o n

Guide to Psychotherapy:
Self-Esteem
http://www.shef.ac.uk/~psysc/psychotherapy/
esteem.htm
Multiple Personality & Dissociative Disorders
http://members.tripod.com/~fsrvival/index.htm

Suggested readings

Applegate M: Multiphasic short-term therapy for dissociative identity disorder, *J Am Psychiatric Nurs Assoc* 3:1, 1997.

Bracken B: Handbook of self-concept, New York, 1996, John Wiley & Sons.

Burns D: Focusing on ego strengths, *Arch Psychiatr Nurs* 5:202, 1991.

Cote I: Current perspectives on multiple personality disorder, *Hosp Comm Psychiatry* 45:827, 1994.

Curtin S: Recognizing multiple personality disorder, *J Psychosoc Nurs Ment Health Serv* 31:29, 1993.

Dallam S, Manderino M: Peer group supports patients with MPD/DD, *J Psychosoc Nurs* 35:22, 1997.

Grame C: Internal containment in the treatment of patients with dissociative disorders, *Bull Menninger Clin* 57:355, 1993.

Kerr N: Ego competency: a framework for formulating the nursing care plan, *Perspect Psychiatric Care* 26:30, 1990.

Kluft R, Fine C: *Clinical perspectives on multiple personality disorder,* Washington, DC, 1993, American Psychiatric Press.

Mruk C: *Self-esteem: research, theory and practice,* New York, 1995, Springer.

Nugent E: Reminiscence as a nursing intervention, *J Psychosoc Nurs* 33:7, 1995.

O'Reilly M: From fragmentation to wholeness: an integrative approach with clients who dissociate, *Perspect Psychiatric Care* 32:5, 1996.

Phillips J: The magic daughter: a memoir of living with multiple personality disorder, New York, 1995, Viking.

Stuart G, Laraia M: *Principles and practice of psychiatric nursing,* ed 6, St Louis, 1998, Mosby.

Vaillant G: *The wisdom of the ego,* Cambridge, Mass, 1993, Harvard University Press.

Emotional Responses and Mood Disorders

Continuum of Emotional Responses

Mood refers to a prolonged emotional state that influences an individual's whole personality and life functioning. It pertains to a person's prevailing and pervading emotion and is synonymous with the terms *affect, feeling state,* and *emotion.* As with other aspects of the personality, emotions or moods serve an adaptive role for the individual. If the expression of emotions is viewed on a continuum of health and illness, the following relevant parameters become apparent (Fig. 12-1):

1. *Emotional responsiveness* involves being affected by and being an active participant in one's internal and external worlds. It implies being open to and aware of one's feelings.
2. *Uncomplicated grief reaction* occurs in response to a loss and implies that a person is facing the reality of the loss and is immersed in the work of grieving.
3. *Suppression of emotions* may be evident as a denial of one's feelings, a detachment from them, or an internalization of all aspects of one's affective world.
4. *Delayed grief reaction* is the persistent absence of any emotional response to a loss. The delay may occur at the start of the mourning process or may become evident later in the process, or both. The delay and rejection of grief may occasionally involve many years.

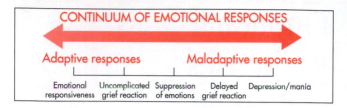

Figure 12-1
Continuum of emotional responses.

5. *Depression,* or melancholia, is an abnormal extension or overelaboration of sadness and grief. It can be used to denote a variety of phenomena: a sign, symptom, syndrome, emotional state, reaction, disease, or clinical entity.
6. *Mania* is characterized by an elevated, expansive, or irritable mood. *Hypomania* is used to describe a clinical syndrome similar to but not as severe as that described by the term *mania* or *manic episode.*
7. Box 12-1 presents facts about depressive and bipolar (manic-depressive) disorders.

Assessment

Behaviors

The behaviors associated with depression are varied (Box 12-2). Sadness and slowness may predominate, or states of agitation may occur. The key element to a behavioral assessment is *change*—the individual changes the usual behavioral pattern and responses. The essential feature of mania is a distinct period of intense psychophysiological activation. Box 12-3 lists some behaviors associated with mania.

Predisposing Factors

Various theories have been proposed to explain severe disturbances of mood. The range of causative factors, which may operate singly or in combination, is evident in the following theories and models:

1. *Genetic factors* have been proposed to account for the transmission of affective disorders through heredity and family history.

Box 12-1   Facts About Mood Disorders

Major Depressive Disorder

- Major depression is among the most common of all clinical problems encountered by primary care practitioners.
- Major depression accounts for more bed days (people off work and in bed) than any other "physical" disorder except cardiovascular disease. Depression is more costly to the economy than chronic respiratory illness, diabetes, arthritis, or hypertension.
- Psychotherapy alone helps some depressed patients, especially those with mild to moderate symptoms.
- Depression can be treated successfully with antidepressant medications in 65% of patients.
- Treatment success rates increase to 85% when alternative or adjunctive medications are used or psychotherapy is combined with medications.

Bipolar (Manic-Depressive) Disorder

- Without modern treatments, patients with bipolar disorder typically spend one-fourth their adult life in the hospital and one-half their life disabled.
- Effective medications (lithium, anticonvulsants), often used in combination with supportive psychotherapy, allow 75% to 80% of manic-depressive patients to lead essentially normal lives.
- These drugs have saved the U.S. economy more than $40 billion since 1970: $13 billion in direct treatment costs and $27 billion in indirect costs.

2. *Aggression-turned-inward theory* suggests that depression results from the turning of angry feelings inward against the self.
3. *Object loss theory* refers to the traumatic separation of a person from significant objects of attachment.
4. *Personality organization theory* describes how a negative self-concept and low self-esteem influence a person's belief system and appraisal of stressors.

Box 12-2 Behaviors Associated with Depression

Affective

Anger
Anxiety
Apathy
Bitterness
Dejection
Denial of feelings
Despondency
Guilt
Helplessness
Hopelessness
Loneliness
Low self-esteem
Sadness
Sense of worthlessness

Physiological

Abdominal pain
Anorexia
Backache
Chest pain
Constipation
Dizziness
Fatigue
Headache
Impotence
Indigestion
Insomnia
Lassitude
Menstrual changes
Nausea
Overeating
Sexual nonrespon-
   siveness
Sleep disturbances
Vomiting
Weight change

Cognitive

Ambivalence
Confusion
Inability to concentrate
Indecisiveness
Loss of interest and motivation
Pessimism
Self-blame
Self-deprecation
Self-destructive thoughts
Uncertainty

Behavioral

Aggressiveness
Agitation
Alcoholism
Altered activity level
Drug addiction
Intolerance
Irritability
Lack of spontaneity
Overdependency
Poor personal hygiene
Psychomotor retar-
   dation
Social isolation
Tearfulness
Underachievement
Withdrawal

Box 12-3   Behaviors Associated with Mania

Affective

Elation or euphoria
Expansiveness
Humor
Inflated self-esteem
Intolerance of criticism
Lack of shame or guilt

Cognitive

Ambition
Denial of realistic danger
Distractibility
Flight of ideas
Grandiosity
Illusions
Lack of judgment
Loose associations

Physiological

Dehydration
Inadequate nutrition
Need for little sleep
Weight loss

Behavioral

Aggression
Excessive spending of
   money
Grandiose acts
Hyperactivity
Increased motor activity
Irresponsibility
Irritability or argumenta-
   tiveness
Poor personal grooming
Provocation
Sexual overactivity
Social activity
Verbosity

5. *Cognitive model* proposes that depression is a cognitive problem dominated by one's negative evaluation of oneself, one's world, and one's future.
6. *Learned helplessness model* suggests that trauma per se does not produce depression, but rather the belief that one has no control over the important outcomes in one's life; therefore the person refrains from making adaptive responses.
7. *Behavioral model* is derived from the social-learning theory framework, which assumes the cause of depression resides in the individual's lack of positively reinforcing interactions with the environment.
8. *Biological model* describes the chemical changes in the body that occur during depressed states, including the deficiency of catecholamines, endocrine dysfunction, hypersecretion of

cortisol neurotransmitter dysregulation, and periodic variations in biological rhythms.

Precipitating Stressors

Four major sources of stressors can precipitate a disturbance of mood, as follows:

1. *Loss of attachment,* real or imagined, includes the loss of love, a person, physical functioning, status, or self-esteem. Because of the actual and symbolic elements involved in the concept of loss, the patient's perception take on primary importance.
2. *Major life events* frequently precede a depressive episode and impact a person's current problems and problem-solving abilities.
3. *Role strain* contributes to the development of depression, particularly in women.
4. *Physiological changes* produced by drugs or various physical illnesses (e.g., infections, neoplasms, metabolic imbalances) can precipitate disturbances of mood. Various antihypertensive drugs and the abuse of addictive substances are common precipitating factors. Most chronic debilitating illnesses are also frequently accompanied by depression. Depression in elderly persons is particularly complex, because the diagnosis often involves evaluating for organic brain damage and clinical depression.

Appraisal of Stressor

Depression results from the interaction among variables at the chemical, experiential, and behavioral levels. The specific form the illness will take depends on the following factors:

1. Genetic vulnerability
2. Developmental events
3. Physiological stressors
4. Psychosocial stressors

This interactive effect underscores the importance of the individual's appraisal of one's life situation and related stressors.

Coping Resources

Coping resources include the person's socioeconomic status, family, interpersonal networks, and the secondary organization provided by the broader social environment. Lack of such personal

Box 12-4   Risk Factors for Depression

Prior episodes of depression
Family history of depression
Prior suicide attempts
Female gender
Age of onset less than 40 years
Postpartum period
Medical comorbidity
Lack of social support
Stressful life events
Personal history of sexual abuse
Current substance abuse

resources provides additional stress for the individual. Box 12-4 lists the risk factors for depression.

Coping Mechanisms

A delayed grief reaction reflects the exaggerated use of the defense mechanisms of denial and suppression in an attempt to avoid the intense distress associated with grief. Depression is similar to abortive grieving, using the mechanisms of repression, suppression, denial, and dissociation. Some believe that mania is a minor image of depression and that, even though the behaviors are dissimilar, the dynamics and coping mechanisms are related.

Nursing Diagnosis

The diagnosis of mood disturbance depends on an understanding of many interrelated concepts, including anxiety, self-concept, and hostility. An appropriate nursing diagnosis should include the patient's maladaptive coping response and related stressor. The box on p. 234 presents the primary and related NANDA nursing diagnoses for maladaptive emotional responses.

Related Medical Diagnoses

The two major categories of mood or affective disorders identified in DSM-IV, bipolar (manic-depressive) disorders and depressive (unipolar) disorders, are based on whether manic and depressive episodes are present over time. In the depressive disorder classifi-

NANDA Nursing Diagnoses Related to Maladaptive Emotional Responses

Anxiety
Communication, impaired verbal
Community coping, ineffective
Coping, ineffective individual
Grieving, anticipatory
*Grieving, dysfunctional
*Hopelessness
Injury, risk for
Loneliness, risk for
Nutrition, altered
Memory, impaired
*Powerlessness
Self-care deficit (specify)
Self-esteem disturbance
Sexual dysfunction
Sleep pattern disturbance
Social isolation
*Spiritual distress
Thought processes, altered
Violence, risk for self-directed

From North American Nursing Diagnosis Association: *NANDA nursing diagnoses: definitions and classification 1997-1998.* Philadelphia, 1997, The Association.
*Primary nursing diagnosis for disturbances in mood.

cation, major depression may involve either a single episode or a recurrent depressive illness but without manic attacks. When the patient has one or more manic episodes, with or without a major depressive episode, the category of bipolar disorder is used. The box on p. 235 describes medical diagnoses related to mood disorders. Box 12-5 lists diagnostic criteria for major depressive and manic episodes.

Outcome Identification

The expected outcome when working with a patient with a maladaptive emotional response is:

The patient will be emotionally responsive and return to preillness level of functioning.

DSM-IV Medical Diagnoses Related to Maladaptive Emotional Responses

DSM-IV Diagnosis	Essential Features
Bipolar I disorder	Current or past experience of a manic episode, lasting at least 1 week, when the person's mood was abnormally and persistently elevated, expansive, or irritable. The episode is sufficiently severe to cause extreme impairment in social or occupational functioning. Bipolar disorders may be classified as manic (limited to only manic episodes), depressed (history of manic episodes with a current depressive episode), or mixed (both manic and depressive episodes).
Bipolar II disorder	Presence or history of one or more major depressive episodes and at least one hypomanic episode. The person has never had a manic episode.
Cyclothymic disorder	History of 2 years of hypomania in which the person experienced numerous periods with abnormally elevated, expansive, or irritable moods. These moods did not meet the criteria for a manic episode, and many periods of depressed mood did not meet the criteria of a major depressive episode.
Major depressive disorder	Presence of at least five symptoms during the same 2-week period, with one being either depressed mood or loss of interest or pleasure. Other symptoms might include weight loss, insomnia, psychomotor agitation or retardation, fatigue, feelings of worthlessness, diminished ability to think, and recurrent thoughts of death. Major depressions may be classified as a single episode or recurrent.
Dysthymic disorder	At least 2 years of a usually depressed mood and at least one of the symptoms mentioned for major depression without meeting the criteria for a major depressive episode.

Modified from American Psychiatric Association: *Diagnostic and statistical manual of mental disorders*, ed 4 (DSM-IV), Washington, DC, 1994, The Association.

Box 12-5 Diagnostic Criteria for Major Depressive and Manic Episodes

Major Depressive Episode

At least five of the following (including one of the first two) must be present most of the day, almost daily, for at least 2 weeks.

1. **Depressed mood**
2. **Loss of interest or pleasure**
3. Weight loss or gain
4. Insomnia or hypersomnia
5. Psychomotor agitation or retardation
6. Fatigue or loss of energy
7. Feelings of worthlessness
8. Impaired concentration
9. Thoughts of death or suicide

Manic Episode

At least three of the following must be present to a significant degree for at least 1 week.

1. Grandiosity
2. Decreased need for sleep
3. Pressured speech
4. Flight of ideas
5. Distractibility
6. Psychomotor agitation
7. Excessive involvement in pleasurable activities without regard for negative consequences

Planning

In care planning the nurse's priorities are the reduction and ultimate removal of all the patient's maladaptive emotional responses, restoration of the patient's occupational and psychosocial functioning, improvement in the patient's quality of life, and minimization of the likelihood of relapse and recurrence. To achieve this, treatment consists of three phases: (1) acute, (2) continuation, and (3) maintenance (Fig. 12-2).

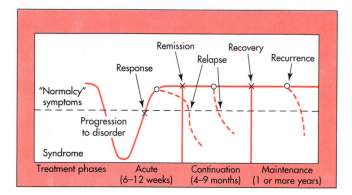

Figure 12-2
Phases of treatment for patients with mood disorders.

Acute

The goal of acute treatment is to eliminate the symptoms. If patients improve with treatment, they have had a *response.* A successful acute treatment brings patients back to an essentially symptom-free state and to a level of functioning comparable to before the illness. This phase usually lasts 6 to 12 weeks, and if patients are symptom free at the end of that time, they are in *remission.*

Continuation

The goal of continuation treatment is to prevent *relapse,* which is the return of symptoms. The risk of relapse is very high in the first 4 to 6 months after recovery, and one of the greatest mistakes in the treatment of mood disorders is the failure to continue a successful treatment for sufficient time. This phase usually lasts 4 to 9 months.

Maintenance

The goal of maintenance treatment is to prevent the *recurrence,* or return, of a new episode of illness. This concept is commonly accepted for bipolar illness but is relatively new for major depressive disorders. Several research studies indicate the effectiveness of maintenance therapy in preventing new depressive episodes or lengthening the interval between them.

A Patient Education Plan for enhancing social skills is presented on p. 238.

Patient Education Plan
Enhancing Social Skills

Content	Instructional Activities	Evaluation
Describe behaviors interfering with social interactions.	Instruct patient on corrective behaviors.	Patient identifies problematic and more facilitative behaviors.
Discuss components of social performance relevant to patient's situation.	Model effective interpersonal skills for patient.	Patient describes specific skills to acquire.
Analyze how patient could incorporate these specific skills.	Use role playing and guided practice to allow patient to test new behaviors.	Patient shows beginning skill in new social behaviors.
Encourage patient to test new skills in other situation.	Give homework assignments for patient to do in natural environment.	Patient discusses ability to complete assigned tasks.
Discuss generalization of new skills to other aspects of patient's life and functioning.	Give feedback, encouragement, and praise for newly acquired social skills and their generalization.	Patient is able to integrate new social behaviors in interactions with others.

Implementation

Intervening in Depression and Mania

Nursing interventions must reflect the complex nature of the integrative model of mood disturbances and address all maladaptive aspects of a patient's life. Intervening in as many areas as possible should have the greatest effect. A Nursing Treatment Plan Summary for patients with maladaptive emotional responses is presented on pp. 240-245.

NURSE ALERT.   In caring for the patient with a severe mood disorder, the nurse should give highest priority to the potential for suicide. Hospitalization is definitely indicated for the patient at risk for suicide. In the presence of rapidly progressing symptoms and in the absence or rupture of the usual support systems, hospitalization is strongly indicated. Nursing care in this case means protecting and assuring patients that they will not be allowed to harm themselves. Patients are at particular risk for suicide when they appear to be coming out of depression; they may then have the energy and opportunity to commit suicide. Acute manic states are also life threatening.

Evaluation

1. Were all possible sources of precipitating stress and the patient's perception of them explored?
2. Was the patient appropriately assessed for problems related to self-concept, anger, and interpersonal relationships?
3. Were changes in the patient's usual behavioral patterns and responses explored?
4. Was the patient's personal and family history of previous episodes of depression or elation fully evaluated?
5. Were appropriate precautions taken for possible suicide or self-harm?
6. Was the patient's social network supported as a coping resource?

Text continued on p. 246

Nursing Treatment Plan Summary
Maladaptive Emotional Responses

Nursing Diagnosis: Hopelessness

Expected Outcome: Patient will be emotionally responsive and return to preillness level of functioning.

Short-term Goals	Interventions	Rationale
Patient's environment will be safe and protective.	Continually evaluate patient's potential for suicide. Hospitalize patient at risk for suicide. Assist patient to move to a new environment when appropriate (e.g., new job, peer group, family setting).	All patients with severe mood disturbances are at high risk for suicide; environmental changes can protect patient, decrease immediate stress, and mobilize additional resources.
Patient will establish a therapeutic relationship with nurse.	Use a warm, accepting, empathic approach. Be aware of and in control of own feelings and reactions (e.g., anger, frustration, sympathy).	Both depressed and manic patients resist becoming involved in a therapeutic alliance; acceptance, persistence, and limit setting are necessary.

With depressed patient:
  Establish rapport through shared time and supportive companionship.
  Allow patient time to respond.
  Personalize care as a way of indicating patient's value as a human being.

With manic patient:
  Give simple, truthful responses.
  Be alert to possible manipulation.
  Set constructive limits on negative behavior.
  Use a consistent approach by all health team members.
  Maintain open communication and sharing of perceptions among team members.
  Reinforce patient's self-control and positive aspects of patient behavior.

Continued

Nursing Treatment Plan Summary

Maladaptive Emotional Responses—cont'd

Short-term Goals	Interventions	Rationale
Patient will be physiologically stable and able to meet self-care needs.	Assist patient to meet self-care needs, particularly in areas of nutrition, sleep, and personal hygiene. Encourage patient's independence whenever possible. Administer prescribed medications and somatic treatments.	Physiological changes occur with disturbances of mood; physical care and somatic therapies are required to overcome these problems
Patient will be able to recognize and express emotions related to daily events.	Respond empathically with a focus on feelings rather than facts. Acknowledge patient's pain and convey a sense of hope in recovery. Help patient experience feelings and then express them appropriately. Assist patient in adaptive expression of anger.	Patients with severe mood disturbances have difficulty identifying, expressing, and modulating feelings.

Patient will evaluate thinking and correct faulty or negative thoughts.

Review patient's conceptualization of the problem but do not necessarily accept conclusions.

Identify patient's negative thoughts and help decrease them.

Help increase positive thinking.

Examine the accuracy of perceptions, logic, and conclusions.

Identify misperceptions, distortions, and irrational beliefs.

Help patient move from unrealistic to realistic goals.

Decrease importance of unattainable goals.

Limit amount of patient's negative personal evaluations.

These strategies help increase patient's sense of control over goals and behaviors, enhance self-esteem, and modify negative expectations.

Continued

Nursing Treatment Plan Summary
Maladaptive Emotional Responses—cont'd

Short-term Goals	Interventions	Rationale
Patient will implement two new behavioral coping strategies.	Assign appropriate action-oriented therapeutic tasks.	Successful behavioral performance counteracts feelings of helplessness and hopelessness.
	Encourage activities gradually, escalating them as patient's energy is mobilized.	
	Provide a tangible, structured program when appropriate.	
	Set goals that are realistic, relevant to patient's needs and interests, and focused on positive activities.	
	Focus on present activities, not past or future activities.	
	Positively reinforce successful performance.	
	Incorporate physical exercise in patient's plan of care.	

Patient will describe rewarding social interactions.	Assess patient's social skills, supports, and interests.	Socialization is an experience incompatible with withdrawal and increases self-esteem through the social reinforcers of approval, acceptance, recognition, and support.
	Review existing and potential social resources.	
	Instruct and model effective social skills.	
	Use role playing and rehearsal of social interactions.	
	Give feedback and positive reinforcement of effective interpersonal skills.	
	Intervene with families to have them reinforce patient's adaptive emotional responses.	
	Support or engage in family and group therapy when appropriate.	

7. Were the nursing interventions broad in scope and inclusive of the many aspects of the patient's world?
8. Were the patient's transference reactions identified and worked through?
9. Was the nurse aware of personal feelings, conflicts, and ability to confront the range of emotions openly throughout the therapeutic relationship?
10. Is the patient experiencing increased satisfaction and pleasure?

your **INTERNET**
c o n n e c t i o n

Internet Depression Resources List
http://www.execpc.com/~corbeau/
Pendulum's Bipolar Disorder/Manic Depression Page
http://www.pendulum.org/

Suggested readings

Beck A et al: *Cognitive therapy of depression,* New York, 1979, Guilford.

Beeber LS: Depression in women. In McBride AB, Austin JK, editors: *Psychiatric–mental health nursing: integrating the behavioral and biological sciences,* Philadelphia, 1996, WB Saunders.

Copeland M: *Living without depression and manic depression: a workbook for maintaining mood stability,* Oakland CA, 1994, New Harbinger Publications.

Depression Guideline Panel: *Depression in primary care,* vol 1, *Detection and diagnosis, Clinical practice guideline,* no 5, pub no 93-0550, Rockville, Md, 1993, US Department of Health and Human Services, Public Health Service, Agency for Health Care Policy and Research.

Depression Guideline Panel: *Depression in primary care,* vol 2, *Treatment of major depression, Clinical practice guideline,* no 5, pub no 93-0551, Rockville, Md, 1993, US Department of Health and Human Services, Public Health Service, Agency for Health Care Policy and Research.

Glod CA: Recent advances in the pharmacotherapy of depression, *Arch Psychiatr Nurs* 10:355, 1996.

Gullette ECD, Blumenthal JA: Exercise therapy for the prevention and treatment of depression, *Pract Psychiatry Behav Health* 9:263, 1996.

Hauenstein E: A nursing practive paradigm for depressed rural women, *Arch Psychiatric Nurs* 11:37, 1997.

Heifner C: The male experience of depression, *Perspect Psychiatric Care* 33:10, 1997.

Jamison K: *An unquiet mind,* New York, 1995, Alfred A Knopf.

Kendall-Tackett K, Kantor G: *Postpartum depression: a comprehensive approach for nurses,* Newbury Park, Calif, 1993, Sage.

Manning M: *Undercurrents: a therapist's reckoning with depression,* San Francisco, 1994, HarperCollins.

Masching J: A nurse battling with her own depression, *J Psychosoc Nurs* 34:26, 1996.

Maynard C: Psychoeducational approach to depression in women, *J Psychosoc Nurs Ment Health Serv* 31:9, 1993.

McEnany G: Rhythm and blues revisited: biological rhythm disturbances in depression, *J Am Psychiatr Nurs Assoc* 2:15, 1996.

NIH Consensus Development Conference: *Diagnosis and treatment of depression in late life,* Rockville, Md, 1991, US Department of Health and Human Services, Public Health Service, National Institutes of Health.

Pollack L: Striving for stability with bipolar disorder despite barriers, *Arch Psychiatric Nurs* 9:122, 1995.

Rosenthal N: *Winter blues: seasonal affective disorder,* New York, 1993, Guilford.

Schwartz A, Schwartz R: *Depression theories and treatments,* New York, 1993, Columbia University Press.

Seligman M: *Learned optimism,* New York, 1991, Knopf.

Shea N et al: The effects of an ambulatory collaborative practice model on process and outcome of care for bipolar disorder, *J Am Psych Nurs Assoc* 3:49, 1997.

Simmons-Alling S: Bipolar mood disorders: brain, behavior, and nursing. In McBride AB, Austin JK, editors: *Psychiatric–mental health nursing: integrating the behavioral and biological sciences,* Philadelphia, 1996, WB Saunders.

Stuart G, Laraia M: *Principles and practice of psychiatric nursing,* ed 6, St Louis, 1998, Mosby.

Suri R, Burt V: The assessment and treatment of postpartum psychiatric disorders, *J Pract Psychiatry Behav Health* 3:67, 1997.

Thase M: Do we really need all these new antidepressants? Weighing the options, *J Pract Psychiatry Behav Health* 3:3, 1997.

Webster D, McEnany G: Research and clinical strategies for treatment resistant depression: buyer beware?, *J Am Psych Nurses Assoc* 3:17, 1997.

Self-Protective Responses and Suicidal Behavior

Continuum of Self-Protection Responses

Self-destructive behavior is any activity that will lead to death if not interrupted. It may be classified as direct or indirect. *Direct self-destructive behavior* includes any form of suicidal activity. The intent is death, and the individual is aware of this as the desired outcome. The behavior is short term in duration. *Indirect self-destructive behavior* includes any activity that is detrimental to a person's physical well-being and that can lead to death. The person is unaware of this potential and usually denies it if confronted. The behavior is usually longer in duration than suicidal behavior. Indirect self-destructive behaviors include the following:

1. Cigarette smoking
2. Driving recklessly
3. Gambling
4. Criminal activity
5. Participating in high-risk recreational activities
6. Substance abuse
7. Socially deviant behavior
8. Stress-seeking behavior
9. Eating disorders
10. Noncompliance with medical treatment

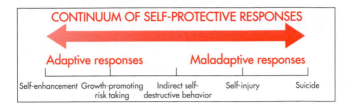

Figure 13-1
Continuum of self-protective responses.

A continuum of self-protecting responses would have self-enhancement as the most adaptive response, with indirect self-destructive behavior, self-injury, and suicide as maladaptive responses (Fig. 13-1).

Assessment

Behaviors

Noncompliance

It has been estimated that half of patients do not comply with their health-care treatment plan. People who do not comply with recommended health-care activities are generally aware that they have chosen not to care for themselves. Box 13-1 lists the most prominent behaviors associated with noncompliance.

Self-injury

Various terms have been used to describe self-injurious behavior: *self-abuse, self-directed aggression, self-harm, self-inflicted injury,* and *self-mutilation.* Self-injury can be defined as the act of deliberate harm to one's own body. The injury is done to oneself, without the aid of another person, and the injury is severe enough for tissue damage. Common forms of self-injurious behavior include cutting and burning the skin, banging head and limbs, picking at wounds, and chewing fingers.

Suicidal behavior

All suicidal behavior is serious, whatever the intent. In the assessment of suicidal behavior, much emphasis is placed on the lethality of the method threatened or used. Although all suicide

Box 13-1 Behaviors Associated with Treatment Noncompliance

Awareness of a reason for noncompliance

Minimization of the seriousness of the problem

Chronic illnesses that are characterized by asymptomatic intervals

Frequent changes in health-care providers

Search for miracle cures

Guilt that interferes with obtaining regular care

Concern about control

threats and attempts must be taken seriously, more vigorous and vigilant attention is indicated when the person is planning or tries a highly lethal means, such as a gunshot, hanging, or jumping. Less lethal means include carbon monoxide and drug overdose, which allow time for discovery once the suicidal action has begun.

Assessment of the suicidal person also includes whether the person has made a specific plan and whether the means to carry out the plan are available. The most suicidal person is one who plans a violent death, has a specific plan, and has the means readily available.

Suicidal behavior is usually divided into the following three categories:

1. *Suicide threats*—a verbal or nonverbal warning that a person is considering suicide. Suicidal persons may indicate verbally that they will not be around much longer or may communicate nonverbally by giving away prized possessions, revising a will, and so on. These messages should be considered in the context of current life events. The threat represents the person's ambivalence about dying. Lack of a positive response may be interpreted as encouragement to carry out the act.

2. *Suicide attempts*—any self-directed actions taken by the individual that will lead to death if not interrupted.

3. *Completed suicide*—may take place after warning signs have been missed or ignored. Persons who make suicide attempts

and who do not really intend to die may do so if they are not discovered in time.

> **NURSE ALERT.** Directly questioning the patient about suicidal thought and plans will not result in the patient taking suicidal actions. Rather, most people will feel relieved to be asked about these feelings. One of the most important questions to ask suicidal patients is whether they think they can control their behavior and refrain from acting on their impulses. If they cannot do this, immediate psychiatric hospitalization is indicated.

Predisposing Factors

Five domains of predisposing factors contribute to understanding self-destructive behavior over the life cycle, as follows:

1. *Psychiatric diagnosis.* More than 90% of adults who end their lives by suicide have an associated psychiatric illness. Three psychiatric disorders that put individuals at particular risk for suicide are mood disorders, substance abuse, and schizophrenia.
2. *Personality traits.* The three aspects of personality that are most closely associated with increased risk of suicide are hostility, impulsivity, and depression.
3. *Psychosocial milieu.* Recent bereavement, separation or divorce, early loss, and decreased social supports are important factors related to suicide.
4. *Family history.* A family history of suicide is a significant risk factor for self-destructive behavior.
5. *Biochemical factors.* Data suggest that serotonergically, opiatergically, and dopaminergically mediated processes may be implicated in self-destructive behavior.

Precipitating Stressors

Self-destructive behavior may result from almost any stress the individual feels is overwhelming. Precipitants are often humiliating life events, such as interpersonal problems, public embarrassment, loss of a job, or the threat of incarceration. In addition, knowing

Box 13-2 Factors in the Assessment of the Self-Destructive Patient

Circumstances of an Attempt

Precipitating humiliating life event
Preparatory actions: acquiring a method, putting affairs in order, suicidal talk, giving away prized possessions, suicidal note
Use of violent method or more lethal drugs/poisons
Understanding of lethality of chosen method
Precautions taken against discovery

Presenting Symptoms

Hopelessness
Self-reproach, feelings of failure and unworthiness
Depressed mood
Agitation and restlessness
Persistent insomnia
Weight loss
Slowed speech, fatigue, social withdrawal
Suicidal thoughts and plans

Psychiatric Illness

Previous suicide attempt
Mood disorders
Alcoholism or substance abuse
Conduct disorders and depression in adolescents
Early dementia and confusional states in elderly schizophrenia
Combinations of the above

Psychosocial History

Recently separated, divorced, or bereaved
Living alone
Unemployed, recent job change or loss
Multiple life stresses (move, early loss, breakup of important relationship, school problems, threat of disciplinary crisis)
Chronic medical illness
Excessive drinking or substance abuse

Box 13-2   Factors in the Assessment of the Self-
Destructive Patient—cont'd

Personality Factors

Impulsivity, aggressivity, hostility
Cognitive rigidity and negativity
Hopelessness
Low self-esteem
Borderline or antisocial disorder

Family History

Family history of suicidal behavior
Family history of mood disorder, alcoholism, or both

---

someone who attempted or committed suicide or being exposed to
suicide through the media may also make the individual more
vulnerable to self-destructive behavior. Box 13-2 lists factors that
the nurse must consider in the assessment of a self-destructive
patient.

Appraisal of Stressor

Suicide prediction is not possible at any meaningful level.
Therefore the nurse must asses each individual for known suicidal
risk factors (Box 13-3) and determine the meaning of each of these
elements for potential suicidal behavior.

Coping Resources

Patients with chronic, painful, or life-threatening illnesses may
engage in self-destructive behavior. Frequently these people
consciously choose to kill themselves. Quality of life becomes an
issue that overrides quantity of life. An ethical dilemma may arise
for nurses who become aware of the patient's choice to engage in
this behavior. No easy answers are available on how to resolve this
conflict. Nurses must do so according to their own belief systems.

Coping Mechanisms

Ego defense mechanisms related to indirect self-destructive behavior are (1) denial, the most prominent coping mechanism,
(2) rationalization, (3) intellectualization, and (4) regression.

Box 13-3 Suicide Risk Factors

Psychosocial and Clinical

Hopelessness
White race
Male gender
Advanced age
Living alone

History

Prior suicide attempts
Family history of suicide attempts
Family history of substance abuse

Diagnostic

General medical illness
Psychosis
Substance abuse
Mood disorders

Defense mechanisms should not be challenged without offering alternative means of coping. They may be standing between the person and suicide.

Suicidal behavior indicates the imminent failure of the coping mechanisms. A suicidal threat may be one last effort to obtain sufficient help to be able to cope. Completed suicide represents the failure of the coping and adaptive mechanisms.

Nursing Diagnosis

The diagnosis of self-destructive behavior must be based on consideration of the seriousness and immediacy of the patient's harmful activity. Patient denial of the self-destructive nature of the behavior must not be allowed to persuade the nurse to underestimate the need for nursing intervention. The nursing diagnosis is related to the nurse's observations combined with data collected by other health-care providers and the information provided by the patient and significant others.

A complete nursing diagnosis is individualized and related to the total constellation of the patient's behaviors and nursing needs.

NANDA Nursing Diagnoses Related to Self-Protective Responses

Adjustment impaired
Anxiety
Body image disturbance
Community coping, ineffective
Coping, ineffective individual
Denial, ineffective
Loneliness, risk for
*Noncompliance (specify)
Self-esteem disturbance
*Self-mutilation, risk for
Spiritual distress
*Violence, risk for: self-directed

From North American Nursing Diagnosis association: *NANDA nursing diagnoses: definitions and classification 1997-1998,* Philadelphia, 1997, The Association.
*Primary nursing diagnosis for self-destructive behavior.

The box above presents the primary and related NANDA nursing diagnoses for maladaptive self-protective responses.

Related Medical Diagnoses

Several medical diagnostic classifications include actual or potential self-destructive behavior among the defining criteria. Suicidal behavior is not separately identified as a diagnostic category. Therefore this section includes medical diagnoses in which this type of behavior is listed as possible. (See Chapter 12 for additional descriptions of the mood disorders.) The disorders included in this section are described in the *Diagnostic and Statistical Manual of Mental Disorders,* fourth edition (DSM-IV), and are identified in the box on p. 256.

Outcome Identification

The expected outcome when working with a patient with maladaptive self-protection responses is:

The patient will not inflict physical self-injury.

DSM-IV Medical Diagnoses Related to Self-Protective Responses

DSM-IV Diagnosis	Essential Features
Bipolar disorder	Presence of a manic episode and no past depressive episodes (see Chapter 12).
Major depressive disorder	Presence of at least five symptoms almost daily during the same 2-week period, with one being either depressed mood or loss of interest or pleasure (see Chapter 12).
Noncompliance with treatment	Noncompliance with an important aspect of treatment for a mental disorder or a general medical condition.
Schizophrenia	Presence of two or more of the following symptoms for a 1-month period: delusions, hallucinations, disorganized speech, disorganized behavior, and negative symptoms (see Chapter 14).
Substance use disorders	Presence of substance dependence or substance abuse (see Chapter 17).

Modified from American Psychiatric Association: *Diagnostic and statistical manual of mental disorders*, ed 4 (DSM-IV), Washington, DC, 1994, The Association.

Planning

The nursing care plan for the person with self-destructive behavior must focus first on protecting the patient from harm. In addition, the plan must address the factors that contributed to the patient's dangerous behavior. The planning process also involves providing the patient with education about the specific illness. A Patient Education Plan for a patient who is noncompliant with medical treatment is presented on p. 258.

NURSE ALERT.   Patients identified as suicidal require special attention from the nurse, who should remember the following guidelines:
1. Take all threats of suicide, verbal or nonverbal, seriously. Report them immediately and institute safety measures.
2. Remove potentially harmful objects from the patient's immediate environment.
3. If the patient is at high risk for suicide, observe constantly, even when the patient is in bed or using the bathroom.
4. Observe carefully when the patient is taking medication. Check the patient's mouth to ensure that pills have been swallowed. Give medication in liquid form if possible.
5. Explain all safety measures to the patient. Communicate caring and concern.
6. Be particularly wary if the patient suddenly becomes calmer and seems at peace. A suicide plan may have been finalized, resulting in relief of anxiety.

Implementation

Intervening in Self-Destructive Behavior

The highest priority nursing interventions are those that protect the patient from immediate danger. In addition, the patient requires assistance in increasing self-esteem and regulating emotions and

Patient Education Plan
Compliance Counseling

Content	Instructional Activities	Evaluation
Assess patient's knowledge of self-care activities.	Ask patient to describe usual lifestyle, diet, exercise, and medication patterns.	Patient describes usual behavior.
	Do described behaviors match self-care instruction received in the past?	Patient repeats previous directions.
Identify areas in which patient behavior differs from healthy self-care practices.	Describe healthy self-care behavior to patient.	Patient discusses problems with compliance.
	Provide written patient education materials.	
	Encourage patient to describe reasons for not performing recommended self-care.	
Discuss alternative approaches to self-care.	Assist patient to identify alternative and more acceptable self-care behaviors.	Patient decides on different approach, shares feelings related to illness.
	Enable patient to talk about feelings related to illness and treatment.	
Agree on a reward for compliant behavior.	Ask patient about reward for practicing good self-care.	Patient identifies reward.
Reinforce new behavior.	Praise patient for making commitment to healthier lifestyle.	Patient recognizes renewed commitment to self-care.

behaviors. The involvement of family and community support systems is recommended. A Nursing Treatment Plan Summary for patients with maladaptive self-protective responses is presented on pp. 260 and 261.

Evaluation

1. Have threats to the patient's physical integrity or self-system been reduced in nature, number, origin, or timing?
2. Do the patient's behaviors reflect concern for own physical, psychological, and social well-being?
3. Have the patient's coping resources been adequately assessed and mobilized?
4. Does the patient describe self and behavior accurately and objectively?
5. Is the patient using adaptive coping responses?
6. Does the patient engage in self-enhancing activities?
7. Is the patient taking reasonable risks that promote personal growth?

Nursing Treatment Plan Summary
Maladaptive Self-Protective Responses

Nursing Diagnosis: Potential for self-directed violence
Expected Outcome: Patient will not inflict physical self-injury.

Short-term Goals	Interventions	Rationale
Patient will not engage in self-injury activities.	Observe closely. Remove harmful objects. Provide a safe environment. Provide for basic physiological needs. Contract for safety if appropriate. Monitor medications.	Highest priority is given to life-saving patient care activities. Patient's behavior must be supervised until self-control is adequate for safety.
Patient will identify positive aspects of self.	Identify patient's strengths. Encourage patient to participate in activities that patient likes and does well. Encourage good hygiene and grooming. Foster healthy interpersonal relationships.	Self-destructive behavior reflects underlying depression related to low self-esteem and anger directed inward.

Patient will implement two adaptive self-protective responses.	Facilitate awareness, labeling, and expression of feelings. Assist patient to recognize unhealthy coping mechanisms. Identify alternative means of coping. Reward healthy coping behaviors.	Maladaptive coping mechanisms must be replaced with healthy ones to manage stress and anxiety.
Patient will identify two social support resources that can be helpful.	Assist significant others to communicate constructively with patient. Promote healthy family relationships. Identify relevant community resources. Initiate referrals to community resources.	Social isolation leads to low self-esteem and depression, perpetuating self-destructive behavior.
Patient will be able to describe the treatment plan and its rationale.	Involve patient and significant others in care planning. Explain characteristics of identified health-care needs, nursing care needs, medical diagnosis, and recommended treatment and medications. Elicit response to nursing care plan. Modify plan based on patient feedback.	Understanding of, and participation in, health-care planning enhance compliance.

Suggested readings

Barstow D: Self-injury and self-mutilation, *J Psychosoc Nurs* 33:19, 1995.

Bultema J: Healing process for the multidisciplinary team: recovering post-inpatient suicide, *J Psychosoc Nurs* 32:19, 1994.

Cardell R, Horton-Deutsch S: A model for assessment of inpatient suicide potential, *Arch Psychiatr Nurs* 8:366, 1994.

Chiles J, Strohsall R: *The suicidal patient: principles of assessment, treatment, and case management,* Washington, DC, 1995, American Psychiatric Press.

Constantino R, Bricker P: Nursing postvention for spousal survivors of suicide, *Issues Ment Health Nurs* 17:131, 1996.

Egan M et al: The "no suicide contract" helpful or harmful? *J Psychosoc Nurs* 35:31, 1997.

Faye P: Addictive characteristics of the behavior of self-mutilation, *J Psychosoc Nurs* 33:36, 1995.

Green J, Grindel C: Supervision of suicidal patients in adult inpatient psychiatric units in general hospitals, *Psychiatric Serv* 47:859, 1996.

Loughrey L et al: Patient self-mutilation: when nursing becomes a nightmare, *J Psychosoc Nurs* 35:30, 1997.

Oxley S, Meter S: The assessment and management of the suicidal patient, *J Pract Psychiatry Behav Health* 1:327, 1996.

Pawlicki C, Gaumer C: Nursing care of the self-mutilating patient, *Bull Menninger Clin* 57:380, 1993.

Rickelman B, Houfek J: Toward an interactional model of suicidal behaviors: cognitive rigidity, attributional style, stress, hopelessness and depression, *Arch Psychiatric Nurs* 9:158, 1995.

Rosenbluth M, Kleinman I, Lowy F: Suicide: the interaction of clinical and ethical issues, *Psychiatr Serv* 46:919, 1995.

Shaffer D: Preventing suicide in young people, *Innovations Research* 2:3, 1993.

Stuart G, Laraia M: *Principles and practice of psychiatric nursing,* ed 6, St Louis, 1998, Mosby.

Werth J: Rational suicide? Implications for mental health professionals, New York, 1996, Taylor & Francis.

Neurobiological Responses and Schizophrenia and Psychotic Disorders

14

Continuum of Neurobiological Responses

The symptoms of psychosis are clustered within five major categories of brain function: cognition, perception, emotion, behavior, and socialization (also referred to as relational). Fig 14-1 presents the continuum of responses related to neurobiological functioning.

Assessment

Behaviors

Schizophrenia is a serious, persistent brain disease that results in psychotic behavior, concrete thinking, and difficulties in information processing, interpersonal relationships, and problem solving. Box 14-1 presents information on how schizophrenia impacts the individual and society.

Related to cognition

Behaviors related to problems in information processing associated with schizophrenia are often referred to as *cognitive defi-*

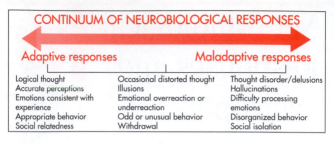

Figure 14-1
Continuum of neurobiological responses.

Box 14-1   Impact of Schizophrenia on the Individual and Society

- About one in every 100 people in the United States (2.5 million) has schizophrenia, regardless of race, ethnic group, or gender.
- In three of four patients, schizophrenia begins between ages 17 and 25.
- Ninety-five percent of patients with schizophrenia have it for their lifetime.
- The cost of family caregiving and crime-related and welfare-related expenditures resulting from schizophrenia is $33 billion annually in the United States.
- More than 75% of taxpayer dollars spent on treatment of mental illness is used for patients with schizophrenia.
- Patients with schizophrenia occupy 25% of all inpatient hospital beds.
- An estimated one third to one half of homeless people in the United States have schizophrenia.
- Schizophrenia is ranked fourth in the top 10 diseases worldwide in terms of burden of illness. The top three are unipolar depression, alcohol use, and bipolar disorder.

Box 14-1   Impact of Schizophrenia on the Individual and Society—cont'd

- Schizophrenia is a chronic illness, five times more common than multiple sclerosis, six times more common than insulin-dependent diabetes, 60 times more common than muscular dystrophy, and 80 times more common than Huntington's disease.
- Of patients with schizophrenia, 25% do not respond adequately to traditional antipsychotic medication.
- From 20% to 50% of patients with schizophrenia attempt suicide; 10% succeed.

cits. They include problems with all aspects of memory, attention, form and content of speech, decision making, and thought content (Box 14-2). Table 14-1 summarizes behaviors related to these problems.

Related to perception

Perception refers to identification and initial interpretation of a stimulus based on information received through the five senses. Box 14-3 summarizes behaviors related to problems with perception. Table 14-2 presents sensory modalities involved in hallucinations.

Related to emotion

Emotions can be hyperexpressed or hypoexpressed in an incongruent manner. Individuals with schizophrenia typically have problems related to hypoexpression (Box 14-4). These patients also often experience emotions related to the difficulties caused by their illness, such as frustration over barriers to accomplishment of personal goals.

Related to movement and behavior

Maladaptive neurobiological responses cause behaviors that are odd, unsightly, confusing, difficult to manage, and puzzling to others (Box 14-5).

Box 14-2 Problems in Cognitive Functioning

Memory

Difficulty retrieving and using stored memory
Impaired short-term/long-term memory

Attention

Difficulty maintaining attention
Poor concentration
Distractibility
Inability to use selective attention

Form and Content of Speech (Formal Thought Disorder)

Loose associations
Tangential/illogical content
Incoherence/word salad/neologism
Circumstantial approach
Pressured/distractible speech
Paucity of speech

Decision Making

Failure to abstract
Indecisiveness
Lack of insight
Impaired concept formation
Impaired judgment
Illogical thinking
Lack of planning and problem-solving skills
Difficulty initiating tasks

Thought Content

Delusions
    Paranoid
    Grandiose
    Religious
    Somatic
    Nihilistic
    Thought broadcasting
    Thought insertion
    Thought control

Table 14-1   Behaviors related to cognitive problems in schizophrenia

Cognitive Problems	Behaviors
Memory	Forgetfulness
	Disinterest
	Lack of compliance
Attention	Difficulty completing tasks
	Difficulty concentrating on work
Form and content of speech	Difficulty communicating thoughts and feelings
Decision making	Difficulty initiating and completing activities
	Concrete thought:
	Inability to carry out multi-stage commands
	Problems with time management
	Difficulty managing money
	Literal interpretation of words and symbols
Thought content	Delusions

Box 14-3   Behaviors Related to Perceptual Problems Associated with Maladaptive Neurobiological Responses

Hallucinations
Illusions
Sensory integration problems
Poor visceral pain recognition
Problems with stereognosis (recognition of objects by touch)
Problems with graphesthesia (recognition of letters "drawn" on the skin)
Misidentification of faces (including self)

Table 14-2 Sensory modalities involved in hallucinations

Sense	Characteristics
Auditory	Hearing noises or sounds, usually in the form of voices. Sounds may range from a simple noise or voice, to a voice talking about the patient, to complete conversations between two or more people about the hallucinating patient. Additional types include audible thoughts, in which the patient hears voices that are speaking what the patient is thinking, commands that tell the patient to do something, sometimes harmful or dangerous.
Visual	Visual stimuli in the form of flashes of light, geometric figures, cartoon figures, and elaborate and complex scenes or visions. Visions can be pleasant or terrifying (e.g., seeing monsters).
Olfactory	Putrid, foul, and rancid smells of a repulsive nature, such as blood, urine, or feces. Occasionally the odors can be pleasant. Olfactory hallucinations are typically associated with stroke, tumor, seizures, and the dementias.
Gustatory	Putrid, foul, and rancid tastes of a repulsive nature, such as blood, urine, or feces.
Tactile	Experiencing pain or discomfort with no apparent stimuli. Feeling electrical sensations coming from the ground, inanimate objects, or other people.
Cenesthetic	Feeling body functions, such as blood pulsing through veins and arteries, food digesting, or urine forming.

Box 14-4 Emotional Responses Occurring in Schizophrenia

Alexithymia—difficulty naming and describing emotions
Apathy—lack of feelings, emotions, interests, or concern
Anhedonia—inability or decreased ability to experience pleasure, joy, intimacy, and closeness

Box 14-5   Abnormal Movements and Behaviors in Schizophrenia

Movements

Catatonia, waxy flexibility, posturing
Extrapyramidal side effects of psychotropic medications
Abnormal eye movements
Grimacing
Apraxia (difficulty carrying out a complex task)
Echopraxia (purposeless imitation of others' movements)
Abnormal gait
Mannerisms

Behaviors

Deterioration in appearance
Aggression/agitation
Repetitive or stereotyped behavior
Avolition (lack of energy and drive)
Lack of persistence at work or school

Box 14-6   Behaviors Associated with Socialization Resulting from Maladaptive Neurobiological Responses

Social withdrawal and isolation
Low self-esteem
Social inappropriateness
Disinterest in recreational activities
Gender identity confusion
Stigma-related withdrawal by others
Decreased quality of life

Associated with socialization

Socialization is the ability to form cooperative and interdependent relationships with others. Box 14-6 summarizes behaviors associated with the relational consequences of maladaptive neurobiological responses.

Finally, the symptoms or behaviors related to schizophrenia have been grouped or categorized in various ways. One prominent

1. *Positive Symptoms*
   Delusions
   Hallucinations
   Thought disorders
   Disorganized speech
   Bizarre behavior

2. *Negative Symptoms*
   Flat affect
   Alogia
   Avolition/apathy
   Anhedonia/asociality
   Attention deficit

5. *Social/Occupational Dysfunction*
   Work/activity
   Interpersonal relationships
   Self-care
   Mortality/morbidity

3. *Cognitive Symptoms*
   Impaired attention
   Impaired memory
   Impaired executive functions
     Abstraction
     Concept formation
     Problem solving
     Decision making

4. *Mood Symptoms*
   Dysphoria
   Suicidal ideation
   Hopelessness

Figure 14-2
Core symptom clusters in schizophrenia.

system groups them into "positive" (additional behaviors) and "negative" (deficit of behaviors) symptoms. Figure 14-2 presents five core symptom clusters that reflect the full impact this illness can have on the individual and society.

Predisposing Factors

Biological

Various neurodevelopmental abnormalities associated with mal-adaptive neurobiological responses are only beginning to be understood, as indicated by the following studies:

1. Brain imaging studies have begun to reveal widespread involvement of the brain in the development of schizophrenia. Lesions in the frontal, temporal, and limbic areas are related to psychotic behaviors. Enlarged ventricles and decreased cortical mass indicate brain atrophy.

2. Several brain chemicals have been implicated in schizophrenia. Research points most strongly to the following:
   - An excess of the neurotransmitter dopamine

- An imbalance between dopamine and other neurotransmitters, especially serotonin
- Problems in the dopamine receptor systems

3. Family studies involving twins and adopted children have suggested a genetic role for schizophrenia. Identical twins, even when raised separately, have a higher co-occurrence of schizophrenia than nonidentical pairs of siblings. Recent genetic research focuses on gene mapping in families with a higher incidence of schizophrenia in first-degree relatives compared with the general population.

Psychological

Psychodynamic theories for the development of maladaptive neurobiological responses have not been supported by research. Unfortunately, earlier psychological theories led to families being blamed for these disorders. This results in families lacking trust in mental health professionals.

Sociocultural

Accumulated stress may contribute to the onset of schizophrenia and other psychotic disorders but is not believed to be the primary cause.

Precipitating Stressors

Biological

Biological stressors related to maladaptive neurobiological responses include (1) interference in the brain's communication and feedback loop, which regulate information processing, and (2) abnormal gating (nerve communication involving electrolytes) mechanisms in the brain, resulting in inability to attend to stimuli selectively.

Environmental

A biologically determined threshold for stress tolerance interacts with environmental stressors to determine the occurrence of disturbed behavior.

Symptom triggers

Triggers are precursors and stimuli that often precede a new episode of illness. Box 14-7 lists common triggers of maladaptive neurobiological responses related to the individual's health, environment, attitudes, and behaviors.

Box 14-7   Symptom Triggers of Maladaptive Neurobiological Responses

Health

Poor nutrition
Lack of sleep
Out-of-balance circadian rhythms
Fatigue
Infection
Central nervous system drugs
Lack of exercise
Barriers to accessing health care

Environment

Hostile or critical environment
Housing difficulties (unsatisfactory housing)
Pressure to perform (loss of independent living)
Changes in life events and daily patterns of
    activity
Interpersonal difficulties
Disruptions in interpersonal relationships
Social isolation and lack of social support
Job pressures (poor occupational skills)
Poverty
Lack of transportation (resources)
Stigmatization

Attitudes/Behaviors

"Poor me" (low self-concept)
"It's hopeless" (lack of self-confidence)
"I'm a failure" (loss of motivation to use skills)
"I have no control" (demoralization)
"No one likes me" (unable to meet spiritual needs)
Feeling overpowered by symptoms
Looks and acts different from others of same age and
    culture
Poor social skills
Aggressive behavior
Violent behavior
Poor medication management
Poor symptom management

Appraisal of Stressor

No scientific research indicates that stress causes schizophrenia. However, studies of relapse and symptom exacerbation provide evidence that stress, the person's appraisal of the stressor, and problems with coping may predict the return of symptoms. The *stress diathesis model* states that schizophrenic symptoms develop based on the relationship between the amount of stress a person experiences and an internal stress tolerance threshold. This is an important model because it integrates biological, psychological, and sociocultural factors in explaining the development of schizophrenia.

Coping Resources

Individual coping resources must be assessed with an understanding of the behavioral results of the brain disorder. Strengths may include such assets as high intelligence or creativity. Parents must actively teach children and young adults coping skills because they cannot usually learn them from observation alone. Family resources may include knowledge about the illness, adequate finances, availability of time and energy, and ability to provide ongoing support.

Coping Mechanisms

Behaviors that represent efforts to protect the patient from the frightening experiences associated with maladaptive neurobiological responses include the following:

- *Regression,* related to information-processing problems and efforts to manage anxiety, leaving little energy for activities of daily living
- *Projection,* as an effort to explain confusing perceptions
- *Withdrawal*

Nursing Diagnosis

The box on p. 274 presents the primary and related NANDA nursing diagnoses for maladaptive neurobiological responses. A complete nursing assessment would include all maladaptive responses, and many additional nursing problems would be identified.

Related Medical Diagnoses

Maladaptive neurobiological responses are included in the medical diagnostic category of schizophrenia and psychotic disorders. The box on pp. 275-277 describes these disorders.

NANDA Nursing Diagnoses Related to Maladaptive Neurobiological Responses

Adjustment, impaired
Anxiety
Caregiver role strain, risk for
*Communication, impaired verbal
Coping family: potential for growth
Coping, ineffective family: compromised
Coping, ineffective individual
Management of therapeutic regimen, individual or family: effective or ineffective
Personal identity disturbance
Role performance, altered
Self-care deficit (bathing/hygiene, dressing/grooming)
Self-esteem disturbance
*Sensory/perceptual alterations (specify)
*Social interaction, impaired
*Social isolation
*Thought processes, altered

From North American Nursing Diagnosis Association: *NANDA nursing diagnoses: definitions and classification 1997-1998,* Philadelphia, 1997, The Association.
*Primary nursing diagnosis for maladaptive neurobiological responses.

O u t c o m e   I d e n t i f i c a t i o n

The expected outcome when working with a patient with maladaptive neurobiological responses is:

The patient will live, learn, and work at the maximum possible level of success, as defined by the individual.

P l a n n i n g

A Family Education Plan for understanding psychosis is presented on pp. 278-280.

Text continued on p. 281

DSM-IV Medical Diagnoses
Related to Maladaptive Neurobiological Responses

DSM-IV Diagnosis	Essential Features
Schizophrenia	At least two of the following, each present for a significant time during a 1-month period:
	1. Delusions
	2. Hallucinations
	3. Disorganized speech
	4. Grossly disorganized or catatonic behavior
	5. Negative symptoms (i.e., flat affect, alogia, avolition)
	For a significant time since the onset of the disturbance, one or more major areas of functioning (e.g., work, interpersonal relations, self-care) are greatly below the level achieved before the onset.
	Continuous signs of the disturbance persist for at least 6 months.
Paranoid type	Preoccupation with one or more delusions or frequent auditory hallucinations.
Disorganized type	All the following are prominent: disorganized speech, disorganized behavior, and flat or inappropriate affect; also, does not meet the criteria for catatonic type.

Continued

DSM-IV Medical Diagnoses
Related to Maladaptive Neurobiological Responses—cont'd

DSM-IV Diagnosis	Essential Features
Catatonic type	At least two of the following dominate the clinical picture: motor immobility, as evidenced by catalepsy or stupor; excessive motor activity; extreme negativism or mutism; peculiarities of voluntary movement, as evidenced by posturing, stereotyped movements, prominent mannerisms, or prominent grimacing; echolalia; and echopraxia.
Undifferentiated type	Symptoms meeting the first general criterion for schizophrenia are present, but criteria for other types are not met.
Residual type	Criteria for schizophrenia or any subtype are not met. Continuing evidence of the disturbance is indicated by negative symptoms or attenuated presence of two or more symptoms included in the general criteria.
Schizophreniform disorder	Meets criteria for schizophrenia, and an episode lasts at least 1 month but less than 6 months. "With" or "without" good prognostic features is specified based on at least two of the following: onset of prominent psychotic symptoms within 4 weeks of first noticeable change in behavior or functioning; confusion or perplexity at the height of the psychosis; good premorbid social and occupational functioning; and absence of blunted or flat affect.

Schizoaffective disorder	Interrupted period of illness, including a major depressive episode or manic episode, concurrent with symptoms of schizophrenia. During the same period of illness, delusions or hallucinations have occurred for at least 2 weeks in the absence of prominent mood symptoms. Symptoms of a mood episode are present during a substantial part of the illness. The condition is not caused by substance abuse or a general medical illness.
Delusional disorder	Nonbizarre delusions (i.e., situations that could occur, such as being followed, being poisoned, or having a disease) lasting at least a month. Has never met criteria for schizophrenia. Apart from the impact of the delusion, functioning and behavior are not greatly affected.
Brief psychotic disorder	Presence of at least one of the following: delusions, hallucinations, disorganized speech, and grossly disorganized or catatonic behavior (behaviors are not culturally sanctioned). Duration of 1 day to 1 month, with eventual return to premorbid functioning. Presence (brief reactive psychosis) or absence of marked stressors.
Shared psychotic disorder (folie à deux)	A delusion develops in an individual in the context of a close relationship with someone who already has a delusion. The delusions of those involved are similar in content.

Modified from American Psychiatric Association: *Diagnostic and statistical manual of mental disorders*, ed 4 (DSM-IV), Washington, DC, 1994, The Association.

Family Education Plan
Understanding Psychosis

Content	Instructional Activities	Evaluation
Describe psychosis	Introduce participants and leaders. State purpose of group. Define terminology associated with psychosis.	Participant describes the characteristics of psychosis.
Identify the causes of psychotic disorders.	Present theories of psychotic disorders. Use audiovisual aids to explain brain anatomy, brain biochemistry, and major neurotransmitters.	Participant discusses the relationship between brain anatomy, brain biochemistry, and major neurotransmitters and the development of psychosis.
Define schizophrenia according to symptoms and diagnostic criteria.	Lead a discussion of the diagnostic criteria for schizophrenia. Show a film on schizophrenia.	Participant describes the symptoms and diagnostic criteria for schizophrenia.
Describe the relationship between anxiety and psychotic disorders.	Present types and stages of anxiety. Discuss steps in reducing and resolving anxiety.	Participant identifies and describes the stages of anxiety and ways to reduce or resolve it.

Analyze the impact of living with hallucinations.	Describe the characteristics of hallucinations. Demonstrate ways to communicate with someone who is hallucinating.	Participant demonstrates effective ways to communicate with a person who has hallucinations.
Analyze the impact of living with delusions.	Describe types of delusions. Demonstrate ways to communicate with someone who has delusions. Discuss interventions for delusions.	Participant demonstrates effective ways to communicate with a person who has delusions.
Discuss the use of psychotropic medications and the role of nutrition.	Provide and explain handouts describing the characteristics of psychotropic medications prescribed for schizophrenia.	Participant identifies and describes the characteristics of medications prescribed for self or family member.

Continued

Family Education Plan
Understanding Psychosis—cont'd

Content	Instructional Activities	Evaluation
Describe the characteristics of relapse and the role of compliance with the therapeutic regimen.	Assist participants to describe their own experiences with relapse. Discuss symptom management techniques and the importance of complying with the therapeutic regimen.	Participant describes behaviors that indicate an impending relapse and discusses the importance of symptom management and compliance with the therapeutic regimen.
Analyze behaviors that promote wellness.	Discuss the components of wellness. Relate wellness to the elements of symptom management.	Participant analyzes the effect of maintaining a state of wellness on the occurrence of symptoms.
Discuss ways to cope adaptively while living with psychosis.	Lead a group discussion focused on the daily problems of living with psychosis and on coping behaviors. Propose ways to create a low-stress environment.	Participant describes ways to modify lifestyle to create a low-stress environment.

Implementation

Nursing interventions may include a broad range of psychosocial and psychobiological treatments and are based on the nurse's assessment of the patient's needs and strengths. Significant others are included whenever possible. The major approaches for nursing intervention with patients who have maladaptive neurobiological responses are summarized as follows:

1. *Behavioral strategies.* Table 14-3 presents strategies for nurses working with patients who have psychoses.
2. *Managing delusions.* Box 14-8 presents strategies for working with delusional patients, and Box 14-9 lists barriers to interventions for delusions.
3. *Managing hallucinations.* Box 14-10 outlines strategies for working with patients to help them cope with ongoing hallucinations.
4. *Psychopharmacology.* Antipsychotic medications are described in Chapter 20.
5. *Managing relapse.* Patients and their family members should be informed about how to identify and take action when a relapse is impending. Box 14-11 lists nursing interventions directed toward preventing relapse, and Box 14-12 is a patient guide for potential relapse.
6. *Patient and family education.* Patients and their families are much better able to manage the illness if they are provided with information about diagnosis, medications, current research, and community resources.

A Nursing Treatment Plan Summary for the patient with maladaptive neurobiological responses is presented on pp. 292-296.

Evaluation

To evaluate nursing interventions with patients who have maladaptive neurobiological responses, the following questions may be asked:

1. Is the patient able to describe the behaviors that characterize the onset of a relapse?
2. Is the patient able to identify and describe the medications prescribed, the reason for taking them, frequency of taking them, and possible side effects?

Text continued on p. 290

Table 14-3 Behavioral strategies for patients with psychosis

Core Problem	Nursing Interventions
Anxiety	Teach patient the symptoms related to anxiety.
	Assist patient to identify what triggers anxiety.
	Help patient use symptom management techniques to cope with anxiety.
	Assess if anxiety is a relapse trigger; if so, devise a plan to reduce anxiety while still in the moderate stage.
Depression	Teach patient the symptoms related to depression.
	Help patient use symptom management techniques to cope with depression.
	Assess if depression is a relapse trigger; if so, devise a plan to reduce depression while still in a mild stage, because a high correlation exists between depression and ability to perform activities of daily living.
Inability to learn from experience	Review both positive and negative experiences.
	Identify what was and was not successful in helping patient achieve the desired goal.
Problems with cause-and-effect reasoning	Analyze each experience to determine what went well and what did not.
	Help patient sequence events leading to the outcome in each experience.
	Consider using rehearsal to enact an event before it occurs.
Difficulty assessing passage of time	Teach patient how to use clocks to tell time.
	Teach patient to use environmental cues (e.g., sun going down, certain radio program) to orient self to time of day.
	Assist patient in creating and maintaining a calendar of scheduled activities.

Concrete thinking	Realize patient sees every problem as having one solution. Teach patient to consider other possible solutions to problems. Realize patient frequently thinks there is only one way to do a task. Create alternative methods to approach situations.
Difficulty telling background from foreground information	Teach patient to distinguish between important and unimportant information. Teach patient to focus on only the important information. Help patient learn to avoid or minimize confusion caused by excess stimulation from noise, large crowds, etc.
Slowed information processing	Give patient time to process and respond to information Minimize anxiety, which increases information-processing difficulties.
Difficulty screening information to share	Demonstrate genuine interest in trying to understand what patient is saying. Use clear and simple language when communicating with patient. Teach patient to identify people who patient can talk to about the illness. Teach patient to contact these people when the symptoms are creating problems. Let patient know you understand the illness and are a "safe person" to talk with.

Continued

Table 14-3 Behavioral strategies for patients with psychosis—cont'd

Core Problem	Nursing Interventions
Communication difficulties	Use active listening to understand patient.
	Clarify what patient is trying to convey.
	Listen for the theme.
	Seek validation from patient on what is communicated.
	Help patient with vocabulary as needed.
	Use the literal meaning of words.
	Have patient repeat what was heard.
	Help patient understand the words and phrases used.
Problems expressing needs	Assist patient to identify and prioritize needs.
	Assist patient to express needs in ways that others will understand.
	Role-play conversations and practice negotiating with others.
Low self-concept	Help patient identify and maximize strengths and positive characteristics.
	Use role play to handle common situations that patients face.
	Give positive feedback when patient handles a situation well.
	Help problem-solve a negative situation to determine how it could have been better handled.
Forced isolation resulting from stigma	Maximize patient's understanding of the illness.
	Teach patient to minimize stigmatizing behaviors when possible.
	Identify comments that are difficult for patient to confront.
	Teach ways to handle stigma and rude comments.
	Develop concrete humorous comebacks.
	Role-play various situations with nurse being the patient.

Difficulty with perception and interpretation of sensory stimuli	Review problematic situations with patient.
	List and assess the thought processes in interpreting events.
	Help patient reality-test and reframe problematic interpretations.
	Reinforce positive and productive processes.
Poor attention span and difficulty completing tasks	Help patient break tasks into small, sequential steps.
	Help patient keep focused on a single task, a step at a time.
	Do not emphasize completing the task.
	Give directions to patient one step at a time.
Inappropriate social behaviors	Identify patient's thought processes that lead to the behavior.
	Ask patient about the behavior.
	Help correct inaccurate perceptions.
	Help patient identify undesirable outcomes of the behavior.
	Teach appropriate social skills.
Difficulty with decision making	Assist patient to decide on desired outcomes.
	Help patient prioritize goals and categorize them into short term and long term.
	Help patient establish a timeline for attainment of each goal.
	Help patient establish small, concrete steps to achieve desired goals.
	Ensure these small steps are achievable by patient and are congruent with patient's culture and values.

Box 14-8 Strategies for Working with Patients with Delusions

Place the delusion in a time frame and identify triggers.
- Identify all the components of the delusion by placing it in time and sequence.
- Identify triggers that may be related to stress or anxiety.
- If delusions are linked to anxiety, teach anxiety management skills.
- Develop a symptom management program.

Assess the intensity, frequency, and duration of the delusion.
- Help patient dispel fleeting delusions in a short time frame.
- Consider temporarily avoiding fixed delusions, or those endured over time, to prevent them from becoming stumbling blocks in the nurse-patient relationship.
- Listen quietly until there is no need to discuss the delusion.

Identify emotional components of the delusion.
- Respond to patient's underlying feelings rather than illogical nature of the delusions.
- Encourage discussion of patient's fears, anxiety, and anger without assuming the delusion is right or wrong.

Observe for evidence of concrete thinking.
- Determine whether or not patient takes you literally.
- Determine if you and patient are using language in the same way.

Observe speech for symptoms of a thought disorder.
- Determine if patient exhibits a thought disorder (e.g., talking in circles, going off on tangents, easily changing subjects, unable to respond to your attempts to redirect).
- Realize that it may not be the appropriate time to point out discrepancy between fact and delusion.

Box 14-8   Strategies for Working with Patients with Delusions—cont'd

Observe for the ability to use cause-and-effect reasoning accurately.
- Determine if patient can make logical predictions (inductive or deductive) based on past experiences.
- Determine if patient can conceptualize time.
- Determine if patient can access and use recent and long-term memory meaningfully.

Distinguish between description of the experience and facts of the situation.
- Identify false beliefs about real situations.
- Promote patient's ability to reality-test.
- Determine if patient is hallucinating because this will strengthen the delusion.

Carefully question the facts as they are presented and their meaning.
- Talk about the delusion to try and help patient see it is not true.
- Note that if this step is taken before the previous steps are completed, it may reinforce the delusion.

Discuss the delusion and its consequences.
- When intensity of the delusion lessens, discuss the delusion when patient is ready.
- Discuss the consequences of the delusion.
- Allow patient to take responsibility for behavior, daily activities, and decision making.
- Encourage patient's personal responsibility for and participation in wellness and recovery.

Promote distraction as a way to stop focusing on the delusion.
- Promote activities that require attention to physical skills and that will help patient use time constructively.
- Recognize and reinforce healthy and positive aspects of patient's personality.

Box 14-9   Barriers to Successful Intervention for Delusions

1. **Becoming anxious and avoiding the patient**
   This leads to annoyance, anger, a sense of hopelessness and failure, feelings of inadequacy,
   and potential laughing at or discounting of the
   patient.
2. **Reinforcing the delusion**
   Do not agree with the delusion, especially to obtain
   the patient's cooperation.
3. **Attempting to prove the patient is wrong**
   Do not attempt a logical explanation.
4. **Setting unrealistic goals**
   Do not underestimate the power of a delusion and the
   patient's need for it.
5. **Becoming incorporated into the delusional
   system**
   This will cause great confusion for the patient and
   make it impossible to establish boundaries of the
   therapeutic relationship.
6. **Failing to clarify confusion surrounding the
   delusion**
   If the nurse does not clearly understand the complexity
   and many intricacies of the delusion, the delusion will
   become more elaborate.
7. **Being inconsistent in intervention**
   The nurse must firmly adhere to the intervention
   plan. "Try anything" approaches lead to
   inconsistency, and the patient is less able to
   identify reality.
8. **Seeing the delusion first and the patient second**
   Avoid using such phrases as, "The person who thinks
   he's being poisoned."

Box 14-10   Strategies for Working with Patients with Hallucinations

Establish a trusting, interpersonal relationship.
- Remember that if you are anxious or frightened, patient will be anxious or frightened.
- Be patient, show acceptance, and use active listening skills.

Assess for symptoms of hallucinations, including duration, intensity, and frequency.
- Observe for behavioral clues that indicate the presence of hallucinations.
- Observe for clues that identify the level of intensity and duration of the hallucination.
- Help patient record the number of hallucinations experienced each day.

Focus on symptoms and ask patient to describe what is happening.
- Empower patient by helping to understand the symptoms experienced or demonstrated.
- Help patient gain control of the hallucinations, seek helpful distractions, and minimize intensity.

Explore drug and alcohol use.
- Determine if patient is using alcohol or drugs (over-the-counter, prescription, or street drugs).
- Determine if these may be responsible for or may exacerbate the hallucinations.

If patient asks, simply say you are not experiencing the same stimuli.
- Respond by letting patient know what is actually happening in the environment.
- Do not argue with patient about differences in perceptions.
- When a hallucination occurs, do not leave patient alone.

Suggest and reinforce the use of interpersonal relationships as a symptom management technique.
- Encourage patient to talk to someone trusted who will give supportive and corrective feedback.
- Assist patient in mobilizing social supports.

Continued

Box 14-10   Strategies for Working with Patients with Hallucinations—cont'd

Help patient describe and compare current and past hallucinations.
- Determine if there is a pattern to patient's hallucinations.
- Encourage patient to remember when hallucinations first began.
- Pay attention to the content of the hallucination, because it may provide clues for predicting behavior.
- Be especially alert for "command" hallucinations that may "compel" patient to act in a certain way.
- Encourage patient to describe past and present thoughts, feelings, and actions as they relate to hallucinations.

Help patient identify needs that may be reflected in the content of the hallucination.
- Identify needs that may trigger hallucinations.
- Focus on patient's unmet needs, and discuss their relationship to the presence of hallucinations.

Determine impact of patient's symptoms on activities of daily living.
- Provide feedback regarding patient's general coping responses and activities of daily living.
- Help patient recognize symptoms, symptom triggers, and symptom management strategies.

---

3. Does the patient participate in relationships with other people at a level that is comfortable for the patient?
4. Is the patient's family aware of the characteristics of the illness and able to participate in a supportive relationship with the patient?
5. Are the patient and family informed about available community resources, such as rehabilitation programs, mental health-care providers, educational programs, and support groups, and do they use them?

Box 14-11   Nursing Interventions to Prevent Relapse

- Identify symptoms that signal relapse.
- Identify symptom triggers.
- Select symptom management techniques.
- Identify coping strategies for symptom triggers.
- Identify support system for future relapse.
- Document action plan in written form and file with key support people.
- Facilitate patient's integration into family and community.

Box 14-12   Patient Guide for Handling Potential Relapse

1. **Go to a safe environment** with someone who can assist you if help is needed. This person should be able to monitor behavior that indicates the relapse is becoming worse.
2. **Reduce the stress and demands on you.** This includes reducing stimuli. Some people find a quiet room where they can be alone, perhaps with soft music. Consider using relaxation or distraction techniques. A quiet place where you can talk with a person you trust is often helpful.
3. **Take medications** if this is part of your program. Work with your prescriber to determine if medications may be useful to reduce relapse. Medications are most helpful when used in a safe, quiet environment and with stress reduction techniques.
4. **Talk to a trusted person** about what the voices are saying to you or about the thoughts you are having. The person needs to know ahead of time that you will call if you need help.
5. **Avoid negative people** who make such comments as, "You're thinking crazy" or "Stop that negative talk."

Nursing Treatment Plan Summary
Maladaptive Neurobiological Responses

Nursing Diagnosis: Altered thought processes
Expected Outcome: Patient will live, learn, and work at the maximum possible level of success, as defined by the individual.

Short-term Goals	Interventions	Rationale
Patient will participate in brief, regularly scheduled meetings with nurse.	Initiate a nurse-patient relationship contract mutually agreed on by nurse and patient. Schedule brief (5- to 10-minute) frequent contacts with patient. Consistently approach patient at scheduled time. Extend length of sessions gradually based on patient's agreement.	Establishment of a trusting relationship is fundamental to developing open communication. A patient with altered thought processes cannot tolerate extended, intrusive interactions and functions best in a structured environment.

Patient will describe delusions and other altered thought processes.	Demonstrate attitude of caring and concern. Validate the meaning of communications with patient. Assist patient to identify the difference between reality and internal thought processes.	Patients are very sensitive to others' responses to their symptoms. A respectful, interested approach enables patient to discuss unusual and frightening thoughts. Identification of reality by a trusted person is helpful.
Patient will identify and describe the effect of brain disease on thought processes.	Provide information about causes of psychoses. Discuss relationship between patient's behaviors and brain function. Involve significant others in educational sessions.	Understanding physiological basis for altered thought processes assists patient to recognize symptoms and to feel in control of the illness. Significant others can provide support and experience less stigma if they are informed about the illness.

Continued

Nursing Treatment Plan Summary
Maladaptive Neurobiological Responses—cont'd

Short-term Goals	Interventions	Rationale
Patient will identify the signs of impending relapse and describe actions to take to prevent relapse.	Assist patient and significant others to identify behaviors related to altered thought processes that indicate threatened relapse. Identify community resources, and mutually plan actions directed toward prevention of relapse.	Relapse can be predicted if patient and family are alert to warning signs. Early intervention allows patient to be in control of the course of the illness. Family members can be helpful in assisting patient to identify symptoms and in providing support for seeking assistance.
Patient will describe symptom management techniques that are helpful in living with altered thought processes.	Describe symptom management techniques that other patients have used. Ask patient to describe techniques used to manage symptoms. Encourage patient to take control of the illness by using symptom management techniques.	Many patients with psychoses continue to have delusions after the acute phase of the illness has passed. They can function better if they learn ways to manage the symptoms.

Nursing Diagnosis: Social isolation

Expected Outcome: Patient will live, learn, and work at the maximum possible level of success, as defined by the individual.

Patient will engage in a trusting relationship with nurse.	Initiate a nurse-patient relationship contract mutually agreed on by nurse and patient. Establish mutual goals related to social interaction. Establish trust by consistently meeting the elements of the plan and engaging in open and honest communication.	Patients who have maladaptive neurobiological responses often have difficulty trusting others. Difficulty with information processing causes problems interpreting the communication of others.
Patient will discuss personal goals related to social interaction.	Encourage patient to describe current relationship patterns. Discuss past relationship experiences. Identify problems associated with social interaction. Explore goals.	Patient may be unaware of the characteristics of mutually satisfying interpersonal relationships. Honest feedback from nurse can assist patient to identify the reasons for past problems. Knowledge of patient's relationship goals leads to development of realistic behavioral change.

Continued

Nursing Treatment Plan Summary
Maladaptive Neurobiological Responses—cont'd

Nursing Diagnosis: Social isolation
Expected Outcome: Patient will live, learn, and work at the maximum possible level of success, as defined by the individual.

Short-term Goals	Interventions	Rationale
Patient will identify behaviors that interfere with social relationships.	Share observations about patient's behavior in social situations.	Identification of problematic behavior helps patient and nurse target changes.
Patient will practice alternative social behaviors with nurse.	Discuss possible behavioral changes that will facilitate establishment of social relationships. Role-play alternative behaviors. Provide feedback.	Practice helps patient feel comfortable with new behaviors. Feedback provides reinforcement for successful behavioral change.
Patient will select one other person and practice social interaction skills.	Discuss experience of practicing new behavior with another person. Discuss ways of maintaining a relationship.	Patient needs ongoing feedback and support related to maintaining behavioral change.

• *Your* **INTERNET** connection

NARSAD: National Alliance for Research on Schizophrenia and Depression
http://www.mhsource.com/narsad.html
The Schizophrenia Home Page
http://www.schizophrenia.com/

Suggested readings

American Psychiatric Association: Practice guideline for the treatment of patients with schizophrenia, *Am J Psychiatry* 154(suppl):4, 1997.

Chouvardas J: The symbolic and literal in schizophrenic language, *Perspect Psychiatr Care,* 32:20, 1996.

Fox JC, Kane CF: Information processing deficits in schizophrenia. In McBride AB, Austin JK, editors: *Psychiatric–mental health nursing: integrating the behavioral and biological sciences,* Philadelphia, 1996, WB Saunders.

Jensen LH, Kane CF: Cognitive theory applied to the treatment of delusions of schizophrenia, *Arch Psychiatr Nurs* 6:335, 1996.

Landeen J et al: Factors influencing staff hopefulness in working with people with schizophrenia, *Issues Ment Health Nurs* 17:457, 1996.

McCay E, Ryan K, Amey S: Mitigating engulfment: recovery from a first episode of psychosis, *J Psychosoc Nurs* 34:40, 1996.

Murphy MF, Moller MD: Symptom management and relapse prevention: a wellness approach, *Dir Psychiatr Nurs,* 1997 (in press).

Nihart M: Atypical antipsychotics and the pharmacology of olanzapine, *J Am Psychiatric Nurs Assoc* 3:S2, 1997.

Parnas J: New views on the psychopathology of schizophrenia. In *Current approaches to psychosis: diagnosis and management,* Excerpta Medica, Reed Elsevier, 1997.

Perese EF: Unmet needs of persons with chronic mental illness: relationship to their adaptation to community living, *Issues Ment Health Nurs* 18:19, 1997.

Rose LE: Caring for caregivers: perceptions of social support, *J Psychosoc Nurs* 35:18, 1997.

Ruscher S, deWit R, Mazmanian D: Psychiatric patients' attitudes about medication and factors affecting noncompliance, *Psychiatric Serv* 48:82, 1997.

Stuart G, Laraia M: *Principles and practice of psychiatric nursing,* ed 6, St Louis, 1998, Mosby.

Yung, A, et al: Monitoring and care of young people at incipient risk of psychosis, *Schizophrenia Bulletin* 22:283, 1996.

Social Responses and Personality Disorders

15

Continuum of Social Responses

Humans are socially oriented. To achieve satisfaction with life, they must establish positive interpersonal relationships. In a healthy interpersonal relationship the individuals involved are close to each other while maintaining separate identities. The persons also must establish interdependence, which is a balance of dependence and independence in the relationship. Fig. 15-1 presents the continuum of social responses.

Development of Mature Interpersonal Relationships

The capacity for interpersonal relationships develops throughout the life cycle. Table 15-1 presents the major developmental tasks related to interpersonal growth.

Personality disorders are usually recognizable by adolescence or earlier and continue throughout most of adulthood. They are enduring, inflexible, and maladaptive patterns of response that are severe enough to cause either dysfunctional behavior or profound distress. Personality disorders are relatively common in the United States; an estimated 6% to 13% of the general population have these illnesses. However, only one fifth of these people are receiving

CONTINUUM OF SOCIAL RESPONSES

Adaptive responses		Maladaptive responses
Solitude	Loneliness	Manipulation
Autonomy	Withdrawal	Impulsivity
Mutuality	Dependence	Narcissism
Interdependence		

Figure 15-1
Continuum of social responses.

Table 15-1   Developmental tasks related to interpersonal growth

Developmental Stage	Task
Infancy	Establish basic trust
Toddlerhood	Develop autonomy and beginning of independent behavior
Preschool age	Learn to display initiative and a sense of responsibility and conscience
School age	Learn competition, cooperation, and compromise
Preadolescence	Become intimate with same-sex friend
Adolescence	Become intimate with opposite-sex friend and independent from parents
Young adulthood	Become interdependent with parents and friends; marry; have children
Middle adulthood	Learn to let go
Late adulthood	Grieve losses and develop a sense of relatedness to the culture

treatment. At least some of these disorders are also associated with greater mortality resulting from suicide.

Assessment

Behaviors

The behaviors observed in people with personality disorders are characterized by chronic, maladaptive social responses. The *Diagnostic and Statistical Manual of Mental Disorders,* fourth edition (DSM-IV), has grouped the personality disorders into three clusters based on descriptive similarities. Table 15-2 presents a specific classification of interpersonal and behavioral characteristics associated with each of the personality disorders. People with cluster B personality disorders have unique character features that at times make nursing care complicated and difficult. Frequently occurring maladaptive responses of patients with cluster B personality disorders include manipulation, narcissism, and impulsivity; Table 15-3 lists behaviors related to these responses.

Predisposing Factors

A variety of factors may lead to maladaptive social responses. Although much research has been done on disorders that affect interpersonal relationships, no specific conclusions exist about their causes. A combination of factors is probably involved, including the following:

1. *Developmental factors.* Any interference with the accomplishment of the developmental tasks listed in Table 15-1 will predispose a person to maladaptive social responses. Disrupted family systems *may* contribute to the development of these responses. Some believe that persons who have these problems were unsuccessful at separating and individuating themselves from their parents. Family norms may discourage relationships outside the family. Family roles are often blurred. Parental alcoholism and child abuse also predispose the person to maladaptive social responses. Organizations of family members are working with professionals to develop a more accurate picture of the relationship between mental disorder and family stress. This collaborative approach should reduce families being blamed by professionals.

2. *Biological factors.* Genetic factors may contribute to maladaptive social responses. Early evidence suggests involvement of the neurotransmitters in the development of these disorders, but further research is needed.

3. *Sociocultural factors.* Social isolation is a major factor in disturbed relationships. This may result from: transiency; norms discouraging approaching others; or the devaluing of less productive members of society, such as elderly, disabled, and chronically ill persons. Isolation may result from the adoption of norms, behaviors, and value systems that differ

Table 15-2   Classification of personality disorders

Disorder	Characteristics
Cluster A: Odd, Eccentric	
Paranoid	Pervasive, unwarranted mistrust of others, manifested by jealousy, envy, and guardedness
	Hypersensitivity; frequent feelings of being mistrusted and misjudged
	Restricted affect, evidenced by lack of tenderness and poor sense of humor
Schizoid	Inability to form social relationships; absence of warm and tender feelings for others
	Indifference to praise, criticism, and feelings of others
	Apparently little or no desire for social involvement; few, if any, close friends
	Generally reserved, withdrawn, and seclusive; preference for solitary interests or hobbies
	Dull or flat affect; appears cold or aloof
Schizotypal	Various oddities of thought, perception, speech, and behavior
	Possible magical thinking, ideas of reference, paranoid ideation, illusions, depersonalization, peculiarities in word choice, social isolation, and inappropriate affect
Cluster B: Dramatic, Emotional, Erratic, Impulsive	
Antisocial	General disregard for others' right and feelings
	History of persistent antisocial behavior
	Poor school or job performance record
	Inability to maintain close interpersonal relationships, especially a sexually intimate one
	Superficial charm, often with manipulative and seductive behavior

Continued

Table 15-2 Classification of personality disorders—cont'd

Disorder	Characteristics
Borderline	Instability in interpersonal behavior, manifested by intense and unstable relationships
	Impulsive and unpredictable behavior
	Profound, inappropriate shifts in mood and affect
	Poor identity, with uncertainty in such areas as self-image, sexual preference, and values
Histrionic	Lively, dramatic, attention-seeking behavior
	Tantrums and angry outbursts
	Demanding, inconsiderate, egocentric behavior
	Manipulative and divisive behavior
	Seductive or charming behavior; superficial personal attachments
Narcissistic	Exaggerated sense of self-importance, manifested by extreme self-centeredness
	Preoccupation with fantasies involving power, success, wealth, beauty, or love
	No capacity for empathy
	Need for constant admiration and attention
	Manipulative behavior

Cluster C: Anxious, Fearful

Avoidant	Anxiety and fearfulness
	Low self-esteem; hypersensitivity to potential humiliation, rejection, or shame
	Social withdrawal accompanied by longing for close relationships
Dependent	Extreme self-consciousness, with feelings of inadequacy and helplessness
	Dependency in relationships; subordinating own needs and leaving major decisions to others
	Overly passive and compliant
Obsessive compulsive	Inability to express affection
	Overly cold and rigid demeanor
	Preoccupation with rules, trivial details, and other expressions of conformity
	Superior attitude; need to control
	Tendency toward perfection, valuing work more than pleasure or relationships

From *Psychiatric nurse review,* Springhouse, Pa, 1990, Springhouse.

Table 15-3 Behaviors related to maladaptive social responses

Maladaptive Response	Behaviors
Manipulation	Treats others as objects
	Centers relationships around control issues
	Is self-oriented or goal oriented, not oriented to others
Narcissism	Fragile self-esteem
	Constant seeking of praise and admiration
	Egocentric attitude
	Envy
	Rage when others are not supportive
Impulsivity	Inability to plan
	Inability to learn from experience
	Poor judgment
	Unreliability

from the majority culture. Unrealistic expectations for relationships is another factor related to these disorders.

Precipitating Stressors

Precipitating stressors generally involve stressful life events, such as losses, that interfere with the person's ability to relate to others and cause anxiety. They can be grouped into the following two categories:

1. *Sociocultural stressors.* Stress can arise from decreased stability of the family unit and separation from significant others, such as from hospitalization.
2. *Psychological stressors.* Prolonged or extremely intense anxiety coexists with a limited ability to cope. Demands to separate from significant others or failure of others to meet dependency needs may cause high levels of anxiety.

Appraisal of Stressor

The mature person who can participate in healthy interpersonal relationships is still vulnerable to the effects of psychological stress. A person's appraisal of the stressor is critically important in this regard. The pain of either a single loss or a series of losses can be so great that the person avoids future involvements rather than risk more pain. This response is more likely if the person had difficulty with developmental tasks pertinent to relatedness.

Coping Resources

Examples of coping resources related to maladaptive social responses include the following:

- Involvement in a broad network of family and friends
- Relationships with pets
- Use of creativity to express interpersonal stress (e.g., art, music, writing)

Coping Mechanisms

Individuals who have maladaptive social responses use a variety of mechanisms in an effort to cope with anxiety. They relate to two specific types of relationship problems as follows:

1. Coping associated with antisocial personality disorder
   - Projection
   - Splitting
   - Devaluation of others
2. Coping associated with borderline personality disorder
   - Splitting
   - Reaction formation
   - Projection
   - Isolation
   - Idealization of others
   - Devaluation of others
   - Projective identification

Nursing Diagnosis

Maladaptive social responses may lead to a range of specific disorders at various levels of severity. The nurse must assess the nature of the patient's disorder and consider the range of behaviors presented.

The box on p. 306 presents the primary and related NANDA nursing diagnoses for maladaptive social responses. A complete nursing assessment would include all maladaptive responses of the patient, and many additional nursing problems would be identified.

Related Medical Diagnoses

Many medically diagnosed psychiatric disorders involve problems with interpersonal relationships. They range in severity from personality disorders to psychoses. The box on pp. 307 and 308 describes these disorders.

NANDA Nursing Diagnoses Related to Maladaptive Social Responses

Adjustment impaired
Anxiety
Coping, ineffective family
Coping, ineffective individual
Family processes, altered
Loneliness, risk for
Management of therapeutic regimen, individual or
    family: ineffective
Parent/infant/child attachment, risk for altered
*__Personal identity disturbance__
Role performance, altered
*__Self-esteem disturbance__
*__Self-mutilation, risk for__
*__Social interaction, impaired__
Social isolation
Thought processes, altered
*__Violence, risk for__
    Self-directed
    Directed at others

From North American Nursing Diagnosis Association: *NANDA nursing diagnoses: definitions and classification 1997-1998,* Philadelphia, 1997, The Association.
*Primary nursing diagnosis for maladaptive social responses.

Outcome Identification

The expected outcome for a patient with maladaptive social responses is:

The patient will obtain maximum interpersonal satisfaction by establishing and maintaining self-enhancing relationships with others.

Planning

A Patient Education Plan for an impulsive patient is presented on pp. 309 and 310.

DSM-IV Medical Diagnoses Related to Maladaptive Social Responses

DSM-IV Diagnosis	Essential Features
Paranoid personality disorder	Pervasive distrust and suspiciousness of others such that their motives are interpreted as malevolent; beginning in early adulthood and present in a variety of contexts.
Schizoid personality disorder	Pervasive pattern of detachment from social relationships and a restricted range of expression of emotions in interpersonal settings; beginning in early adulthood and present in a variety of contexts.
Schizotypal personality disorder	Pervasive pattern of social and interpersonal deficits marked by acute discomfort with and reduced capacity for close relationships and by cognitive and perceptual distortions and eccentricities of behavior; beginning in early adulthood and present in a variety of contexts.
Antisocial personality disorder	Pervasive patter of disregard for and violation of the rights of others occurring since age 15 years.
Borderline personality disorder	Pervasive pattern of instability in interpersonal relationships, self-image, and affect and marked impulsivity; beginning by early adulthood and present in a variety of contexts.
Histrionic personality disorder	Pervasive pattern of excessive emotionality and attention seeking; beginning by early adulthood and present in a variety of contexts.

Continued

DSM-IV Medical Diagnoses
Related to Maladaptive Social Responses—cont'd

DSM-IV Diagnosis	Essential Features
Narcissistic personality disorder	Pervasive pattern of grandiosity (in fantasy or behavior), need for admiration, and lack of empathy; beginning by early adulthood and present in a variety of contexts.
Avoidant personality disorder	Pervasive pattern of social inhibition, feelings of inadequacy, and hypersensitivity to negative evaluation; beginning by early adulthood and present in a variety of contexts.
Dependent personality disorder	Pervasive and excessive need to be taken care of that leads to submissive and clinging behaviors and fears of separation; beginning by early adulthood and present in a variety of contexts.
Obsessive-compulsive personality disorder	Pervasive pattern of preoccupation with orderliness, perfectionism, and mental and interpersonal control, at the expense of flexibility, openness, and efficiency; beginning by early adulthood and present in a variety of contexts.

Modified from American Psychiatric Association: *Diagnostic and statistical manual of mental disorders*, ed 4 (DSM-IV), Washington, DC, 1994, The Association.

Patient Education Plan
Modifying Impulsive Behavior

Content	Instructional Activities	Evaluation
Describe characteristics and consequences of impulsive behavior.	Select a situation in which impulsive behavior occurred. Ask patient to describe what happened. Instruct patient to keep a diary of impulsive actions, including a description of events before and after the incident.	Patient identifies and describes an impulsive incident. Patient maintains a diary of impulsive behaviors. Patient explores the causes and consequences of impulsive behavior.
Describe behaviors characteristic of interpersonal anxiety; relate anxiety to impulsive behavior.	Discuss the diary with patient. Assist patient to identify interpersonal anxiety related to impulsive behavior.	Patient connects feelings of interpersonal anxiety with impulsive behavior.

Continued

Patient Education Plan
Modifying Impulsive Behavior—cont'd

Content	Instructional Activities	Evaluation
Explain stress reduction techniques.	Describe the stress response. Demonstrate relaxation exercises. Assist patient to return the demonstration.	Patient performs relaxation exercises when signs of anxiety appear.
Identify alternative responses to anxiety-producing situations.	Using situations from the diary and knowledge of relaxation exercises, assist patient to list possible alternative responses. Role-play each of the identified alternative behaviors.	Patient identifies at least two alternative responses to each anxiety-producing situation.
Practice using alternative responses to anxiety-producing situations.	Discuss the feelings associated with impulsive behavior and the alternatives.	Patient describes the relationship between behavior and feelings. Patient selects and performs anxiety-reducing behaviors.

Implementation

The essential elements of nursing intervention with the patient who has maladaptive social responses include the following:

1. Establishing a therapeutic relationship
2. Involving the family to promote and maintain positive change
3. Providing a therapeutic milieu that focuses on realistic expectations, involving the patient in decision making, and processing interactional behaviors in current situations
4. Setting limits and providing structure
5. Protecting the patient from self-harm
6. Focusing on the patient's strengths
7. Implementing contracting and other cognitive-behavioral strategies

A Nursing Treatment Care Plan Summary for the patient who has maladaptive social responses is presented on pp. 312-314.

Evaluation

The following questions may assist the nurse to evaluate the outcomes of intervention with the patient who has maladaptive social responses:

1. Has the patient become less impulsive, manipulative, or narcissistic?
2. Does the patient express satisfaction with the quality of interpersonal relationships?
3. Can the patient participate in close interpersonal relationships?
4. Does the patient verbalize recognition of positive behavioral change?

Nursing Treatment Plan Summary
Maladaptive Social Responses

Nursing Diagnosis: Impaired social interaction

Expected Outcome: Patient will obtain maximum interpersonal satisfaction by establishing and maintaining self-enhancing relationships with others.

Short-term Goals	Interventions	Rationale
Patient will participate in a therapeutic nurse-patient relationship.	Initiate a nurse-patient relationship contract mutually agreed on by patient and nurse. Develop mutual behavioral goals. Maintain consistent behavior by all nursing staff. Communicate honest responses to patient's behavior. Provide honest, immediate feedback about behavioral change. Maintain confidentiality. Demonstrate accessibility.	An atmosphere of trust facilitates open expression of thoughts and feelings, a trusting relationship enables patient to risk sharing feelings; honest responses reinforce openness; staff consistency creates a predictable environment that creates trust.

Goal	Intervention	Rationale
Patient will describe interpersonal strengths and weaknesses.	Provide patient with opportunities to demonstrate strengths (e.g., helping other patients, assuming leadership roles). Assist patient to analyze experiences perceived as failures. Communicate acceptance of patient as a person while not accepting maladaptive social behavior.	Patient with maladaptive social responses is unable to identify accurately interpersonal strengths and weaknesses, leading to fear of closeness and fear of failure. Nurse must assist patient to separate behavioral incidents from total self-worth and to recognize that patient can be liked even if imperfect.
Patient will establish or reestablish one interpersonal relationship that is mutually satisfying and adaptive.	Provide consistent feedback about adaptive and maladaptive social behavior. Encourage patient to describe successful and unsuccessful relationship experiences orally or in a written journal. Assist patient in initiating or resuming a relationship with one other person. Review aspects of this relationship with patient. Reinforce patient's adaptive social responses. Evaluate with patient alternatives to maladaptive social responses.	Describing and evaluating one's behavior require taking responsibility for the behavior and its consequences. Patients need to go beyond understanding or insight to engaging in actual behavioral change. Nurse must help patient evaluate whether responses are adaptive or maladaptive. Alternatives can then be identified to further the patient's goal achievement.

Continued

Nursing Treatment Plan Summary
Maladaptive Social Responses—cont'd

Nursing Diagnosis: High risk for self-mutilation
Expected Outcome: Patient will select constructive rather than self-destructive ways of coping with interpersonal anxiety.

Short-term Goals	Interventions	Rationale
Patient will not engage in self-mutilation	Develop a contract with patient to notify staff when anxiety is increasing.	When patient is not able to cope with anxiety, protecting patient's safety is nurse's highest priority.
	Provide close one-on-one observation of patient when necessary to maintain safety.	
	Remove all potentially dangerous objects from patient and environment.	
	Provide prescribed medications.	
Patient will describe self-mutilating episodes.	Assist patient in reviewing these events.	A contract helps patient assume responsibility and explore healthier coping responses.
	Identify cues and triggers that precede self-mutilating behavior.	Self-mutilation is often a way of relieving extreme anxiety.
	Help patient explore feelings related to these episodes.	Structured interpersonal support can help patient review these events.

Patient will describe alternatives to self-mutilating behaviors.	Suggest alternative behaviors, such as seeking interpersonal support or engaging in an adaptive anxiety-reducing activity.	Nurse can help patient review the full range of adaptive responses. Supportive but critical evaluation is necessary for behavioral change.
Patient will implement one new adaptive response when experiencing high interpersonal anxiety.	Assist patient in selecting new adaptive responses. Reinforce patient's adaptive behavior. Identify positive consequences of the adaptive responses. Discuss ways these may be generalized to other situations.	Nurse should take an active role in setting limits, examining patient behaviors, and reinforcing adaptive actions. These new learned responses can also be reviewed for their applicability to other life events.

your **INTERNET**
c o n n e c t i o n

BPD Central
Borderline Personality Disorder
http://members.aol.com/BPDCentral/index.html
Borderline Personality Disorder Page
http://www.cmhc.com/disorders/sx10t.htm

Suggested readings

Amey S: Transitional objects, phenomena, and relatedness: understanding and working with individuals with borderline personality disorder, *J Am Psychiatric Nurs Assoc* 2:143, 1996.

Derksen J: *Personality disorders: clinical and social perspectives,* New York, 1995, Wiley & Sons.

Dyckoff D et al: The investigation of behavioral contracting in patients with borderline personality disorder, *J Psychiatr Nurs Assoc* 2:71, 1996.

Field S: Milieu-based treatment of the borderline patient: a self psychology perspective, *Continuum* 1(2):133, 1994.

Greene H, Ugarriza D: The 'stably unstable': borderline personality disorder: history, theory, and nursing intervention, *J Psychosoc Nurs* 33:26, 1995.

Hagerty B et al: An emerging theory of human relatedness, *Image* 25:291, 1993.

Hampton M: Dialectical behavior therapy in the treatment of persons with borderline personality disorder, *Arch Psychiatric Nurs* 11:96, 1997.

Henson R: Analysis of the concept of mutuality, *Image* 29:77, 1997.

Link P: *Clinical assessment and management of severe personality disorders,* Washington, DC, 1996, American Psychiatric Press.

Miller B: Characteristics of effective day treatment programming for persons with borderline personality disorder, *Psychiatric Serv* 46:605, 1995.

Miller C, Eisner W, Allport C: Creative coping: a cognitive-behavioral group for borderline personality disorder, *Arch Psychiatr Nurs* 8:280, 1994.

Miller S: Borderline personality disorder from the patient's perspective, *Hosp Community Psychiatry* 12:1215, 1994.

Nehls N: Brief hospital treatment plans for persons with borderline personality disorder: perspectives of inpatient psychiatric nurses and community mental health center clinicians, *Arch Psychiatric Nurs* 8:303, 1994.

Sperry L: *Handbook of diagnosis and treatment of the DSM-IV personality disorders,* New York, 1995, Brunner/Mazel.

Stuart G, Laraia M: *Principles and practice of psychiatric nursing,* ed 6, St Louis, 1998, Mosby.

Cognitive Responses and Organic Mental Disorders

16

Continuum of Cognitive Responses

Models of Cognition

1. *Learning model.* This psychological learning theory states that when an individual experiences a stimulus, several behavioral responses are available. The most likely response is one that has been reinforced in the past.
2. *Social cognitive model.* This psychological learning theory states that a stimulus is experienced as a sign that creates a demand, leading a person to seek gratification. The response is guided by a person's perception of the environment.
3. *Piaget developmental model.* See Table 16-1.

Fig. 16-1 illustrates the continuum of cognitive responses.

Assessment

Behaviors

The specific cognitive disorders to be considered include delirium and dementia. Table 16-2 describes the characteristics of delirium and dementia. Depression in elderly people is often misdiagnosed as dementia and is included in Table 16-2 for purposes of comparison.

Table 16-1 Piaget's levels of cognitive development

Stage	Age (Years)	Characteristics
Sensorimotor	Birth to 2	Action oriented No language Develops awareness of body in space Develops memory for missing objects
Preparation and organization of concrete operations		
Preoperational phase	2 to 5	Appearance of symbolism Objects defined by function Magical thinking
Concrete operations	5 to 12	Capable of relatability Syllogistic (deductive) reasoning Makes and follows rules Quantifies experience
Formal operations	12 to 14 and older	Abstraction Development of ideals Criticism of others Self-criticism

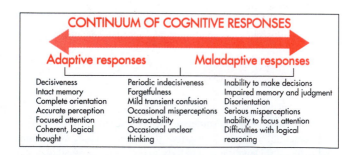

Figure 16-1
Continuum of cognitive responses.

Table 16-2 Comparison of delirium, depression, and dementia

	Delirium	Depression	Dementia
Onset	Rapid (hours to days)	Rapid (weeks to months)	Gradual (years)
Course	Wide fluctations; may continue for weeks if cause not found	May be self-limited or may become chronic without treatment	Chronic; slow but continuous decline
Level of consciousness	Fluctuates from hyperalert to difficult to arouse	Normal	Normal
Orientation	Patient is disoriented, confused	Patient may seem disoriented	Patient is disoriented, confused
Affect	Fluctuating	Sad, depressed, worried, guilty	Labile; apathy in later stages
Attention	Always impaired	Difficulty concentrating; patient may check and recheck all actions	May be intact; patient may focus on one thing for long periods
Sleep	Always disturbed	Disturbed; excess sleeping or insomnia, especially early-morning waking	Usually normal
Behavior	Patient is agitated, restless	Patient may be fatigued, apathetic; may occasionally be agitated	Patient may be agitated or apathetic; may wander
Speech	Sparse or rapid; patient may be incoherent	Flat, sparse, may have outbursts; understandable	Sparse or rapid; repetitive; patient may be incoherent

Continued

Table 16-2   Comparison of delirium, depression, and dementia—cont'd

	Delirium	Depression	Dementia
Memory	Impaired, especially for recent events	Varies day to day; slow recall; often short-term deficit	Impaired, especially for recent events
Cognition	Disordered reasoning	May seem impaired	Disordered reasoning and calculation
Thought content	Incoherent, confused, delusions, stereotyped	Negative, hypochondriac, thoughts of death, paranoid	Disorganized, rich content, delusional, paranoid
Perception	Misinterpretations, illusions, hallucinations	Distorted; patient may have auditory hallucinations; negative interpretation of people and events	No change
Judgment	Poor	Poor	Poor; socially inappropriate behavior
Insight	May be present in lucid moments	May be impaired	Absent
Performance on mental status exams	Poor but variable; improves during lucid moments and with recovery	Memory impaired; calculation, drawing, following directions usually not impaired; frequent "I don't know" answers	Consistently poor; progressively worsens; patient attempts to answer all questions

From Holt J: *Am J Nurs* 93(8):32, 1993.

Predisposing Factors

Cognitive responses are generally the result of a biological disruption in the functioning of the central nervous system (CNS). Factors that predispose the individual to developing cognitive disorders include the following:

1. Interference with the supply of oxygen, glucose, and other essential basic nutrients to the brain
   - Arteriosclerotic vascular changes
   - Transient ischemic attacks
   - Cerebral hemorrhage
   - Multiple small brain infarcts
2. Degeneration associated with aging
3. Collection of toxic substances in brain tissue
4. Alzheimer's disease
5. Human immunodeficiency virus (HIV)
6. Chronic liver disease
7. Chronic renal disease
8. Vitamin deficiencies (particularly thiamine)
9. Malnutrition
10. Genetic abnormalities

Major psychiatric disorders, such as schizophrenia, bipolar disorder, anxiety disorders, and depression, may also influence cognitive functioning.

Precipitating Stressors

Any major assault on the brain is likely to result in a disruption in cognitive functioning. Categories of stressors include the following:

1. Hypoxias
2. Metabolic disorders, including hypothyroidism, hyperthyroidism, hypoglycemia, hypopituitarism, and adrenal disease
3. Toxicity and infection
4. Adverse response to medication
5. Structural changes in the brain, such as tumors or traumas
6. Sensory underload or overload

Appraisal of Stressor

The specific stressor related to cognitive impairment often cannot be identified, although this is rapidly changing as neuroscientific knowledge increases. In general, when assessing maladaptive cognitive responses, physiological causes are ruled out first, then psychosocial stressors are considered. Even when physiological factors are present, psychosocial stress may further compromise the person's thought process. Thus the person's appraisal of the stressor is critically important.

Coping Resources

Individual responses include strengths and skills. Caregivers can be supportive and can also provide information about the person's personality characteristics, habits, and routines. Self-help groups can be effective coping resources for caregivers.

Coping Mechanisms

The way an individual copes emotionally with maladaptive cognitive responses is greatly influenced by past life experience. A person who has developed many coping mechanisms that have been effective in the past is better able to handle the onset of a cognitive problem than a person who already has coping problems. Usual coping mechanisms may be exaggerated as the person tries to adapt to loss of cognitive ability.

Because the basic behavioral disruption in delirium is altered awareness, which reflects a severe biological disturbance in the brain, psychological coping mechanisms are not generally used. For this reason the nurse must protect the patient from harm and substitute for the person's own coping mechanisms by constantly reorienting the patient and reinforcing reality.

Behaviors that may represent attempts by the person with dementia to cope with loss of cognitive ability may include suspiciousness, hostility, joking, depression, seductiveness, and withdrawal.

Ego defense mechanisms that may be observed in patients with cognitive impairment include the following:

- Regression
- Denial
- Compensation

Nursing Diagnosis

Most disorders that result in some degree of cognitive impairment are physiological in origin. Therefore the nurse must consider the patient's physical needs as well as the psychosocial behavioral problems. A thorough nursing diagnosis reflects all these influences on the patient's behavior. If the patient's cognitive disability interferes with participation in the treatment planning process, it may be necessary to involve a significant other in the formation of the nursing diagnosis.

The box below presents the primary and related nursing diagnoses for maladaptive cognitive responses. A complete nursing assessment would include all the patient's nursing care needs, and many additional nursing diagnoses would be identified.

Related Medical Diagnoses

The box on pp. 324 and 325 describes mental disorders that result in maladaptive cognitive responses.

NANDA Nursing Diagnoses Related to Maladaptive Cognitive Responses

Anxiety
Communication, impaired verbal
***Confusion, acute**
***Confusion, chronic**
Coping, ineffective family: compromised
Coping, ineffective individual
***Environmental interpretation syndrome, impaired**
Health maintenance, altered
Home maintenance management, impaired
Incontinence, bowel
Injury, risk for
***Memory, impaired**
Physical mobility, impaired
Role performance, altered
Self-care deficit, bathing/hygiene, dressing/grooming, feeding, toileting
Sensory/perceptual alterations (specify): visual, auditory, kinesthetic, gustatory, tactile, olfactory
Sleep pattern disturbance
Social interaction, impaired
Social isolation
***Thought processes, altered**

From North American Nursing Diagnosis Association: *NANDA nursing diagnoses: definitions and classification 1997-1998*, Philadelphia, 1997, The Association.
*Primary nursing diagnosis for maladaptive cognitive responses.

DSM-IV Medical Diagnoses Related to Cognitive Responses

DSM-IV Diagnosis	Essential Features
Delirium (general criteria) (to be applied to all other categories of delirium)	Disturbed consciousness accompanied by a cognitive change that cannot be accounted for by a dementia.
	Impaired ability to focus, sustain, or shift attention.
	Cognitive changes, including impaired recent memory, disorientation to time or place, language disturbance, or perceptual disturbance.
	Develops over a short time; tends to fluctuate during the course of the day.
Delirium due to a general medical condition	Evidence that the cognitive disturbance is the direct result of a general medical condition.
Substance-induced delirium	Evidence of substance intoxication or withdrawal, medication side effects, or toxin exposure judged to be related to the delirium.
Delirium with multiple etiologies	Evidence of multiple causes for the delirium.
Dementia (general criteria) (to be applied to all other categories of dementia)	Development of multiple cognitive deficits, including memory impairment and at least one of the following: aphasia, apraxia, agnosia, or disturbed executive functioning (ability to think abstractly and plan, initiate, sequence, monitor, and stop complex behavior).
	Must cause severe impairment in social or occupational functioning.
Dementia of the Alzheimer's type	Gradual onset with continuing cognitive decline.
	All other causes of dementia must be ruled out.

Vacular dementia	Focal neurological signs and symptoms or laboratory evidence of cerebrovascular disease that are judged to be related to the dementia.
Dementia due to other general medical conditions	Evidence that the general medical condition (e.g., HIV, traumatic brain injury, Parkinson's disease, Huntington's disease, Pick's disease, Creutzfeldt-Jakob disease, normal-pressure hydrocephalus, hypothyroidism, brain tumor, vitamin B_{12} deficiency) is etiologically related to the dementia.
Substance-induced persisting dementia	Deficits do not occur exclusively during a delirium and persist beyond the usual duration of substance intoxication or withdrawal. Evidence that the deficits are related to persisting effects of substance use (e.g., drug of abuse, medication).
Dementia due to multiple etiologies	Evidence that the dementia has more than one etiology.
Amnestic disorder (general criteria)	Development of memory disorder evidenced by impaired ability to learn new information or to recall previously learned information. Disturbance causes significant impairment in social or occupational functioning and represents a significant decline from a previous level of functioning. Does not occur exclusively during the course of delirium or dementia.
Amnestic disorder due to a general medical condition	Evidence that the disturbance is directly related to a general medical condition (including physical trauma).
Substance-induced persisting amnestic disorder	Evidence that the memory disturbance is etiologically related to the persisting effects of substance use (e.g., drug abuse, medication).

Modified from American Psychiatric Association: *Diagnostic and statistical manual of mental disorders*, ed 4 (DSM-IV), Washington, DC, 1994, The Association.

Outcome Identification

The expected outcome for a patient with maladaptive cognitive responses is:

The patient will achieve optimum cognitive functioning.

Planning

A Family Education Plan for the family of a patient with maladaptive cognitive responses is presented on pp. 327 and 328.

Implementation

Intervening in Delirium

Nursing interventions for the patient with delirium include the following:

> **NURSE ALERT.** Restraining a delirious patient to maintain an intravenous line may increase agitation. Use restraint only when absolutely necessary, and never leave a restrained delirious patient alone.

1. *Meeting physiological needs*
   - Maintain nutrition and fluid/electrolyte balance.
   - Use nursing measures such as back rub, warm milk, and soothing conversation to promote sleep. Sedatives may be contraindicated until the cause of the delirium has been found.
2. *Intervening in perceptual disturbances* (e.g., hallucinations)
   - Keep light on in room to minimize shadows.
   - Ensure safety by placing the patient in a room with security screens and removing excess furniture.
   - Provide one-to-one nursing care if needed to maintain orientation.
   - Reorient frequently to time, place, and person.
3. *Communication*
   - Give clear messages.
   - Avoid giving choices.
   - Use simple, direct statements.

Family Education Plan
Helping a Family Member with Maladaptive Cognitive Responses

Content	Instructional Activities	Evaluation
Explain possible causes of maladaptive cognitive responses.	Describe predisposing factors and precipitating stressors that may lead to impaired cognition; provide printed reference materials.	Family identifies possible causes of patient's disorders.
Define and describe orientation to time, place, and person.	Define three spheres of orientation; role-play interpersonal responses to disorientation.	Family identifies disorientation and provides reorientation.
Describe relationship of cognitive functioning level to ability to communicate.	Describe impact of maladaptive cognitive responses on communication; demonstrate effective communication techniques; videotape and discuss return demonstration.	Family adjusts communication approaches to patient's ability to interact.

Continued

Family Education Plan
Helping a Family Member with Maladaptive Cognitive Responses—cont'd

Content	Instructional Activities	Evaluation
Describe effect of mal-adaptive cognitive responses on self-care behaviors.	Describe usual progression of gain or loss of self-care ability related to nature of disorder; encourage learner to assist in providing care to patient; provide written instructional materials.	Family assists with activities of daily living as required by patient's level of biopsychosocial functioning.
Refer to community resources.	Provide a list of community resources; arrange to meet with staff members of selected community programs; visit meetings of selected programs.	Family describes various programs that provide services relevant to patient's and family's needs and will contact appropriate programs when needed.

4. *Patient education*
   - Provide information regarding cause of delirium.
   - Teach the patient and family about prescribed treatment.
   - Inform about prevention of future episodes.
   - Refer to community health nursing agency if further education or nursing intervention is required.

Intervening in Dementia

Nursing interventions for the patient with dementia include the following:

1. *Orientation*
   - Mark room clearly with the patient's name.
   - Encourage the patient to keep personal possessions in room.
   - Use a night light.
   - Provide clocks and calendars.
   - Provide newspapers and discuss them with the patient.
   - Orient verbally at frequent intervals.
2. *Communication*
   - Introduce yourself.
   - Show unconditional positive regard for the patient.
   - Use clear, concise verbal communication.
   - Modulate voice.
   - Avoid pronouns.
   - Use yes/no questions.
   - Request one thing at a time.
   - Ensure that verbal agrees with nonverbal communication.
   - Learn about the patient's past life.
   - Provide a sense of sheltered freedom.
3. *Reinforcing coping mechanisms*
4. *Decreasing wandering.* Map the patient's behavior to identify conditions under which the behavior occurs, and intervene preventively.
5. *Decreasing agitation*
   - Explain expectations clearly.
   - Offer choices if the patient can handle them.
   - Provide a schedule of activities.
   - Avoid power struggles. If the patient refuses a request, leave and return in a few minutes.
   - Involve the patient in care whenever possible.

6. *Pharmacological approaches.* Tacrine (Cognex) and done-
   pezil (Aricept) delay progression of Alzheimer's disease.
7. *Involving family members*
8. *Using community resources*

Table 16-3 presents a clinical pathway for elderly patients with
cognitive impairment. Nursing interventions with patients who
have maladaptive cognitive responses are provided in the Nursing
Treatment Plan Summary on pp. 334 and 335.

Evaluation

1. Was the assessment complete enough to correctly identify
   the problem?
2. Were the goals individualized for this patient?
3. Was enough time allowed for goal achievement?
4. Did nurse have the skills needed to carry out the identified
   interventions?
5. Did environmental factors affect goal achievement?
6. Did additional stressors affect the patient's ability to cope?
7. Was the goal achievable for this patient?
8. What alternative approaches could be tried?

Table 16-3   Clinical pathway: hospital guide for elderly patients with cognitive impairment

	Preadmission	Day 1	Day 2	Day 3	Day 4	Days 5-7/ Discharge
Consults	Neurology, neuropsychiatric testing	Neurology, medical, neuropsychiatry, VNA/home health				
Tests	SMA 7-12, CBC, VDRL, sedimentation rate, vitamin B_{12} folate, T_3, T_4, TSH; MRI or CT within 6 months; CXR and EEG	Anything not done preadmission	Evaluate laboratory studies; EEG for medication monitoring		Tuberculosis test	
Assessments	Preadmission criteria met; medical records; family/patient interview; patient's support systems, ADLs, and related activities; MMSE, CMAI, CDS, Blessed, ADAS, AIMS	Initial psychiatric evaluation; CDS, MMSE, Behav-AD, WPS; nursing assessment; CMAI for sleep agitation; monitor progress	Complete/repeat scales; monitor treatments; AIMS, CDS, MMSE, WPS	Repeat	Repeat	Repeat

Table 16-3 Clinical pathway: hospital guide for elderly patients with cognitive impairment—cont'd

	Preadmission	Day 1	Day 2	Day 3	Day 4	Days 5-7/ Discharge
Anxiety/safety level	Assess for falls, violence, suicidality, and fears about hospitalization	Order groups: environment, awareness, ADLs, reminiscing, exercise, OT/RT	Engage in groups	Repeat	Repeat	Repeat
Medications	Obtain list of prescriptions and OTCs: doses, purposes, side effects	Evaluate need for PRNs for agitation/sleep	Pharmacologic treatments for identified behavioral/ emotional symptoms	Evaluate for changes in symptoms and medication needs	Repeat	Repeat
Education	Provide family with informational and GeroPsychiatry Program sheets	Evaluate educational needs of patient, family, and caregiver; select a program	Plan family meeting; include interdisciplinary team members	Repeat	Family meeting: health teaching/ aftercare issues	Family meeting: review recall of teaching and reinforce

Special needs	Potential patient needs (e.g., diet, mobility, vision, hearing); discuss GPHP with family	Evaluate for GPHP placement needs at discharge; implement risk protocol for falls	Determine GPHP needs; discuss placement	Repeat	Decide on GPHP; if placed, notify about admission and arrange transportation	Refer for other special needs
Discharge plan	Preliminary discharge needs and date; disposition contract	Discuss finances/community resources with family; make discharge plans	Maintain family contact/involvement	Repeat	Repeat; arrange discharge	Repeat; confirm discharge plans with agencies; assist patient

Data courtesy of Behavioral Intensive Care Unit, Institute of Psychiatry and Behavioral Sciences, Medical University of South Carolina, Charleston, 1997. *VNA,* Visiting Nurses Association; *SMA 7-12,* Sequential Multiple Analyzer for concentrations of total protein, albumin, total bilirubin, alkaline phosphatase, (lactate dehydrogenase, and aspartate aminotransferase; $T_3,$ triiodothyronine; $T_4,$ thyroxine; *TSH,* thyroid-stimulating hormone; *MRI,* magnetic resonance imaging; *CT,* computed tomography; *CXR,* chest x-ray film; *EEG,* electroencephalogram; *ADLs,* activities of daily living; *MMSE,* Mini Mental State Exam; *CMAI,* Cohen Mansfield Agitation Inventory; *CDS,* Cornell Depression Scale; *Blessed,* Blessed Dementia Scale; *ADAS,* Alzheimer's Disease Assessment Scale; *AIMS,* Abnormal Involuntary Movement Scale; *Behav-AD,* Behavioral Pathology in Alzheimer's Disease Rating Scale; *WPS,* Washington Paranoia Scale; *OT/RT,* occupational and recreational therapy; *OTCs,* over-the-counter drugs; *PRNs,* medications prescribed as necessary; *GPHP,* Geriatric Partial Hospitalization Program.

Nursing Treatment Plan Summary
Maladaptive Cognitive Responses

Nursing Diagnosis: Altered thought processes
Expected Outcome: Patient will achieve optimum cognitive functioning.

Short-term Goals	Interventions	Rationale
Patient will meet basic biological needs.	Maintain adequate nutrition; monitor fluid intake and output; monitor vital signs.	Basic biological integrity is necessary for survival.
	Provide opportunities for rest and stimulation.	Interventions related to survival are given high priority for nursing intervention.
	Assist with ambulation if necessary.	
	Assist with hygiene activities as needed.	
Patient will be safe from injury.	Assess sensory and perceptual functioning.	Maladaptive cognitive responses usually involve sensory and perceptual disorders that can endanger patient's safety.
	Provide access to eyeglasses, hearing aids, canes, walkers, etc., if needed.	
	Observe and remove safety hazards (e.g., obstacles, slippery floors, open flames, inadequate lighting).	
	Supervise medications if necessary.	
	Protect from injury during periods of agitation with one-to-one nursing care; use restraints only if absolutely necessary.	

| Patient will experience an optimum level of self-esteem. | Provide reality orientation.
Establish a trusting relationship.
Encourage independence.
Identify interests and skills; provide opportunities to use them.
Give honest praise for accomplishments.
Use therapeutic communication techniques to help patient communicate thoughts and feelings. | Cognitive impairment is a threat to self-esteem; a positive nurse-patient relationship can assist patient to express fears and feel secure in the environment; recognition of accomplishments also raises self-esteem. |
| Patient will maintain positive interpersonal relationships. | Initiate contact with significant others.
Encourage patient to interact with others; involve in group activities.
Teach family and patient about nature of the problem and recommended health care plan.
Allow significant others to assist in patient care.
Meet with significant others regularly and provide them with an opportunity to talk.
Involve patient and family in discharge planning. | Caring relationships with others promote a positive self-concept; communication by significant others can often be understood more easily than that of strangers; family and friends can provide help in knowing patient's habits and preferences; involvement of significant others in caregiving often helps them cope with the stress of patient's health problem. |

your **INTERNET**
c o n n e c t i o n

Alzheimer's Association
http://www.alz.org/

Family Caregiver Alliance
http://www.caregiver.org/text/index.htm

Suggested readings

Abraham IL et al: Multidisciplinary assessment of patients with Alzheimer's disease, *Nurs Clin North Am* 29:113, 1994.

Breitner JCS, Walsh KA: Diagnosis and management of memory loss and cognitive disorders among elderly persons, *Psychiatr Serv* 46:29, 1995.

Colenda C: Managing agitated dementia patients: a decision analysis approach, *J Pract Psychiatry Behav Health* 3:156, 1997.

Fopma-Loy J, Austin J: An attributional analysis of formal caregivers' perceptions of agitated behavior of a resident with Alzheimer's disease, *Arch Psychiatric Nurs* 7:217, 1993.

Grinspoon L, editor: Update on Alzheimer's disease. Part I, *Harvard Ment Health Lett* 11:1, 1995.

Hamdy RC et al: *Alzheimer's disease: a handbook for caregivers,* ed 2, St Louis, 1994, Mosby.

Kolanowski AM: Disturbing behaviors in demented elders: a concept synthesis, *Arch Psychiatr Nurs* 9:188, 1995.

Kumar V, Goldstein MZ, Doraiswamy PM: Advances in pharmacotherapy for decline of memory and cognition in patients with Alzheimer's disease, *Psychiatr Serv* 47:249, 1996.

Li G et al: Age at onset and familial risk in Alzheimer's disease, *Am J Psychiatry* 152:424, 1995.

Liken M, Collins C: Grieving: facilitating the process for dementia caregivers, *J Psychosoc Nurs* 31:21, 1993.

Patkar A, Kunkel E: Treating delirium among elderly patients, *Psychiatric Serv* 48:46, 1997.

Powell L, Courtice K: Alzheimer's disease: a guide for families, Reading, Mass, 1993, Addison-Wesley.

Rentz CA: Reminiscence: a supportive intervention for the person with Alzheimer's disease, *J Psychosoc Nurs Ment Health Serv* 33:15, 1995.

Stuart G, Laraia M: *Principles and practice of psychiatric nursing,* ed 6, St Louis, 1998, Mosby.

Swanson EA, Maas ML, Buckwalter KC: Catastrophic reactions and other behaviors of Alzheimer's residents: special unit compared with traditional units, *Arch Psychiatr Nurs* 7:292, 1993.

Chemically Mediated Responses and Substance-Related Disorders

17

Continuum of Chemically Mediated Responses

Although there is a continuum from occasional drug or alcohol use to frequent use to abuse and dependence, not everyone who uses substances becomes an abuser, and every abuser does not become dependent. **Substance abuse** refers to continued use even after problems occur. **Substance dependence** indicates a severe condition, usually considered a disease. **Addiction** generally refers to the psychosocial behaviors related to substance dependence. The terms *addiction* and *dependence* are often used interchangeably. **Dual diagnosis** refers to the coexistence of substance abuse and psychiatric disorders within the same person. **Withdrawal symptoms** result from a biological need for the drug. **Tolerance** means that it takes increasing amounts of the substance to produce the expected effect. Withdrawal symptoms and tolerance are signs of **physical dependence.**

Abused substances include alcohol, opiates, prescription medications, psychotomimetics, cocaine, marijuana, and inhalants. A serious and growing problem in substance abuse is the rapidly increasing use of more than one substance simultaneously or sequentially.

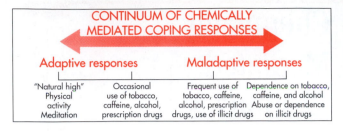

Figure 17-1
Continuum of chemically mediated coping responses.

An individual may achieve a state of relaxation, euphoria, stimulation, or altered awareness by various means. Fig. 17-1 illustrates the range of these activities.

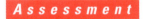

Behaviors

Behaviors that indicate the presence of a substance abuse problem can be assessed by using a screening tool. Box 17-1 presents the Brief Drug Abuse Screening Tool (B-DAST), and Box 17-2 presents the CAGE screening tool for alcoholism. Table 17-1 compares blood alcohol levels and observable behaviors. Table 17-2 summarizes the behaviors associated with substance abuse.

Individuals who abuse substances face other risks because of their lifestyle. Accidents and violence occur frequently. Self-neglect contributes to physical, mental, and dental disease. Intravenous drug users and their partners are at high risk for infections with bloodborne pathogens, including human immunodeficiency virus (HIV) and hepatitis B virus (HBV). Finally, individuals who are dually diagnosed have both a substance use and a psychiatric disorder. Their substance use (1) may be causing the psychopathology; (2) may be secondary to the psychopathology as they self-medicate with substances to treat the symptoms of their mental disorder, use substances to enhance symptoms, or use substances to counter the side effects of medications they are taking for their psychiatric disorder; or (3) may be coincidental and not related to the mental disorder.

Box 17-1   Brief Drug Abuse Screening Test (B-DAST)

Instructions: The following questions concern information about your involvement in and abuse of drugs. Drug abuse refers to (1) the use of prescribed or over-the-counter drugs in excess of the directions and (2) any non-medical use of drugs. Carefully read each statement and decide whether your answer is yes or no. Then circle the appropriate response.

YES NO   1. Have you used drugs other than those required for medical reasons?

YES NO   2. Have you abused prescription drugs?

YES NO   3. Do you abuse more than one drug at a time?

YES NO   4. Can you get through the week without using drugs (other than those required for medical reasons)*?

YES NO   5. Are you always able to stop using drugs when you want to?*

YES NO   6. Have you had blackouts or flashbacks as a result of drug use?

YES NO   7. Do you ever feel bad about your drug abuse?

YES NO   8. Does your spouse (or parents) ever complain about your involvement with drugs?

YES NO   9. Has drug abuse ever created problems between you and your spouse?

YES NO   10. Have you ever lost friends because of your use of drugs?

YES NO   11. Have you ever neglected your family or missed work because of your use of drugs?

*Items 4 and 5 are scored in the "no" or false direction.

Continued

Box 17-1 Brief Drug Abuse Screening Test (B-DAST)—cont'd

YES NO 12. Have you ever been in trouble at work because of drug abuse?
YES NO 13. Have you ever lost a job because of drug abuse?
YES NO 14. Have you gotten into fights when under the influence of drugs?
YES NO 15. Have you engaged in illegal activities in order to obtain drugs?
YES NO 16. Have you ever been arrested for possession of illegal drugs?
YES NO 17. Have you ever experienced withdrawal symptoms as a result of heavy drug intake?
YES NO 18. Have you ever had medical problems as a result of your drug use (e.g., memory loss, hepatitis, convulsions, bleeding)?

YES NO 19. Have you ever gone to anyone for help for a drug problem?
YES NO 20. Have you ever been involved in a treatment program specifically related to drug use?

From Skinner HA: *Addict Behav* 7:363, 1982.

Box 17-2   The CAGE Questionnaire

- Have you ever felt you ought to **C**ut down on your drinking?
- Have people **A**nnoyed you by criticizing your drinking?
- Have you ever felt bad or **G**uilty about your drinking?
- Have you ever had a drink first thing in the morning to steady your nerves or get rid of a hangover (**E**yeopener)?

Scoring: 1 "yes" answer calls for further inquiry.

From Ewing JA: *JAMA* 252:1905, 1984.

Table 17-1   Comparison of blood alcohol concentrations to behavioral manifestations of intoxication

Blood Alcohol Level (g/dl)	Behaviors
0.05 to 0.15	Euphoria, labile mood, cognitive disturbances (decreased concentration, impaired judgment, loss of sexual inhibitions)
0.15 to 0.25	Slurred speech, staggering gait, diplopia, drowsiness, labile mood with outbursts
0.3	Stupor, aggressive behavior, incoherent speech, labored breathing, vomiting
0.4	Coma
0.5	Severe respiratory depression, death

From Antai-Otong D: *Am J Nurs,* vol 95, August 1995.

Predisposing Factors

1. *Biological factors*
   - Familial tendency, especially for alcohol abuse
   - Altered alcohol metabolism resulting in an uncomfortable physiological response
   - Variants of the DRD2 gene, which appears to be associated with the transmission of alcoholism

Table 17-2 Characteristics of substances of abuse

Substance/Common Street Names	Route/Physical Dependence/ Psychological Dependence	Signs and Symptoms	Special Considerations/ Consequence of Use
DEPRESSANTS			
Alcohol Booze, brew, juice, spirits	Ingestion Yes/yes	*Use* Depression of major brain functions such as mood, cognition, attention, concentration, insight, judgment, memory, affect, emotional rapport in interpersonal relationships; extent of depression is dose dependent and ranges from lethargy through anesthesia and death; psychomotor impairment, increased reaction time, interruption of hand-eye coordination, motor ataxia, nystagmus, decreased rapid eye movement sleep leading to more dreams and sometimes nightmares	Chronic alcohol use leads to serious disruptions in most organ systems: malnutrition and dehydration; vitamin deficiency leading to Wernicke's encephalopathy and alcoholic amnestic syndrome; impaired liver function, including hepatitis and cirrhosis; esophagitis, gastritis, pancreatitis; osteoporosis; anemia; peripheral neuropathy; impaired pulmonary function; cardiomyopathy; myopathy; disrupted immune system; brain damage
Barbiturates Barbs, beans, black beauties, blue angels, candy, downers, goof balls, G.B., nebbies, reds, sleepers, yellow jackets, yellows	Ingestion, injection Yes/yes		
Benzodiazepines Downers	Ingestion, injection Yes/yes		

Overdose

Unconsciousness, coma, respiratory depression, death

Withdrawal

General depressant withdrawal syndrome; tremors, agitation, anxiety, diaphoresis, increased pulse and blood pressure, sleep disturbances, hallucinosis, seizures, delusions, delirium tremens (DTs)

Postacute withdrawal: mood swings, difficulty sleeping, impaired cognitive functioning, increased emotionality, overreaction to stress

Low-dose/high-dose benzodiazepine withdrawal:

Low—therapeutic doses for no more than 6 months; subtle symptoms, peak in about 12 days; wax and wane for 6-12 months; several symptoms-free days, followed by acute anxiety, dilated pupils, elevated pulse and blood pressure

High—peaks in 2-3 days for short-acting and 5-8 days for longer-acting drugs; symptoms usually gone in 2 weeks

High susceptibility to other dependencies

Dependence on barbiturates and benzodiazepines may develop insidiously; users may underreport actual amount taken because of guilt about multiple prescriptions and abuse

Continued

Table 17-2 Characteristics of substances of abuse—cont'd

Substance/Common Street Names	Route/Physical Dependence/ Psychological Dependence	Signs and Symptoms	Special Considerations/ Consequence of Use
STIMULANTS			
Amphetamines A, AMT, bam, bennies, crystal, diet pills, dolls, eye openers, lid poppers, pep pills, purple hearts, speed, uppers, wake-ups	Ingestion, injection Yes/yes	**Use** Sudden rush of euphoria, abrupt awakening, increased energy, talkativeness, elation; agitation, hyperactivity, irritability, grandiosity, pressured speech; diaphoresis, anorexia, weight loss, insomnia, increased temperature/blood pressure/pulse, tachycardia, ectopic heart beats, chest pain, urinary retention, constipation, dry mouth *High-dose:* slurred, rapid, incoherent speech; stereotypical movements, ataxic gait, teeth grinding, illogical thought processes, headache, nausea, vomiting *Toxic psychosis:* paranoid delusions in clear sensorium; auditory, visual, or tactile hallucinations; very labile mood, unprovoked violence	Certain amphetamines prescribed for attention deficit hyperactivity disorder in children because of a paradoxical depressant action; may be used alternately with depressants
Cocaine Bernice, bernies, big C, blow, C, charlie, coke, dust, girl, heaven, jay, lady, nose candy, nose pow-	Inhalation, smoking, injection, topical Yes/yes		Cocaine use may lead to multiple physical problems: destruction of the nasal septum related to snorting; coronary artery vasoconstriction; seizures; cerebrovascular accidents; transient ischemic episodes; sudden death related to

der, snow, sugar,
white lady; crack
= conan, freebase,
rock, toke, white
cloud, tornado

Overdose

Seizures, cardiac arrhythmias, coronary artery spasms, myocardial infarction, marked increase in blood pressure and temperature, which can lead to cardiovascular shock and death

Withdrawal

"*Crash*": depression, agitation, anxiety, intense drug craving; followed by fatigue, depression, loss of drug desire, insomnia, desire for sleep; followed by prolonged sleep then extreme hunger, renewed drug cravings, anergia, and anhedonia, which may increase for 1-4 days

Pattern varies widely among patients; anxiety, depression, irritability, fatigue may last several weeks; craving may return; relapse is a risk

Sometimes a user stops stimulants purposely to decrease tolerance, decreasing the amount needed to "get high"

respiratory arrest and
myocardial infarction

Intravenous use of stimulants may lead to the serious physical consequences described under opiates

Intravenous use of stimulants may lead to the serious physical consequences described under opiates

Continued

Table 17-2 Characteristics of substances of abuse—cont'd

Substance/Common Street Names	Route/Physical Dependence/ Psychological Dependence	Signs and Symptoms	Special Considerations/ Consequence of Use
OPIATES			
Heroin H, horse, harry, boy, scag, shit, smack, stuff, white junk, white stuff	Ingestion, smoking, inhalation Yes/yes	*Use* Euphoria, relaxation, relief from pain, nodding out (apathy, detachment from reality, impaired judgment, drowsiness), constricted pupils, nausea, constipation, slurred speech, respiratory depression	Intravenous use leads to high risk for infection with bloodborne pathogens, such as HIV or hepatitis B; other infections (e.g., skin abscesses, phlebitis, cellulitis, and septic emboli causing pneumonia, pulmonary abscess, or subacute bacterial endocarditis) may occur as a result of lack of asepsis or contaminated substances; adulterants (e.g., talc, starch, strychnine) deposited in lungs, causing impaired function
Morphine	Injection		
Meperidine	Injection, ingestion	*Overdose* Unconsciousness, coma, respiratory depression, circulatory depression, respiratory arrest, cardiac arrest, death	
Codeine	Ingestion, injection	Anoxia can lead to brain abscess	
Opium	Smoking, ingestion		
Methadone	Ingestion	*Withdrawal* *Initially:* drug craving, lacrimation, rhinorrhea, yawning, diaphoresis	

In 12-72 hours: sleep disturbances, mydriasis, anorexia, piloerection, irritability, tremor, weakness, nausea, vomiting, diarrhea, chills, fever, muscle spasms (especially in legs), flushing, spontaneous ejaculation, abdominal pain, hypertension, increased rate and depth of respirations
Protracted withdrawal: changes in respirations and temperature, decreased self-esteem, anxiety, depression, drug hunger, abnormal responses to stressful situations; lasts up to 6 months

Chronic use leads to lack of concern about physical well-being resulting in malnutrition and dehydration; criminal behavior may occur to acquire money for drugs
Multiple drug use is common

MARIJUANA

Acapulco gold, aunt mary, broccoli, dope, grass, grunt, hay, hemp, herb, J, joint, joy stick, killer weed, marjane, pot, ragweed, reefer, smoke, weed

Smoking
ingestion
No/yes

Use
Altered state of awareness, relaxation, mild euphoria, reduced inhibition, red eyes, dry mouth, increased appetite, increased pulse, decreased reflexes; panic reaction
Overdose
Toxic psychosis
Withdrawal
None

Pulmonary problems; interference with reproductive hormones; may cause fetal abnormalities

Continued

Table 17-2 Characteristics of substances of abuse—cont'd

Substance/Common Street Names	Route/Physical Dependence/ Psychological Dependence	Signs and Symptoms	Special Considerations/ Consequence of Use
HALLUCINOGENS			
Acid, big D, blotter, blue heaven, cap, D, deeda, flash, L, mellow yellows, microdots, paper acid, sugar, ticket, yello	Ingestion, smoking No/no	*Use* Distorted perceptions and hallucinations in presence of a clear sensorium; distortions of time and space, illusions, depersonalization, mystical experiences, heightened sense of awareness; extreme mood lability; tremor, dizziness, piloerection, paresthesias, synesthesia, nausea and vomiting; increased temperature, pulse, blood pressure, and salivation; panic reaction, "bad trip" *Overdose* Rare with LSD; convulsions, hyperthermia, death *Withdrawal* None	Flashbacks may last for several months; permanent psychosis may occur

PHENCYCLIDINE (PCP)

Angel dust, DOA, dust, elephant, hog, peace pill, supergrass, tic tac

Smoking, ingestion

No/no

Use

Intensely psychotic experience characterized by bizarre perceptions, confusion, disorientation, euphoria, hallucinations, paranoia, grandiosity, agitation; anesthesia; apparent enhancement of strength and endurance, rage reactions; may be agitated and hyperactive with tendency toward violence or catatonic and withdrawn, or vacillate between the two conditions; red, dry skin; dilated pupils, nystagmus, ataxia, hypertension, rigidity, seizures

Overdose

Seizures, coma, death

Withdrawal

None

If flashbacks occur, they are mild and usually not disturbing

Continued

Table 17-2   Characteristics of substances of abuse—cont'd

Substance/Common Street Names	Route/Physical Dependence/ Psychological Dependence	Signs and Symptoms	Special Considerations/ Consequence of Use
INHALANTS			
Spray, rush, bolt, huffing, bagging, sniffing	Inhalation Yes/Yes	*Use* *Psychological:* belligerence, assaultiveness, apathy, impaired judgment *Physical:* dizziness, nystagmus, incoordination, slurred speech, unsteady gait, depressed reflexes, tremor, blurred vision, euphoria, anorexia *Overdose* Lethargy, stupor/coma, respiratory arrest, cardiac arrhythmia *Withdrawal* Headaches, chills, abdominal cramps, delirium tremors (not common)	Death from inhalants can occur in different ways: Sudden death is caused by cardiac arrhythmia—sometimes this happens the first time the child uses inhalants Suicide may be a result of impaired judgment. Injury: under the influence of inhalants youth feel invulnerable Burns and frostbite can also be caused by these chemicals Permanent cognitive impairment may require an individual to reside in a structured setting

2. *Psychological factors*
   - Oral-dependent personality types
   - Low self-esteem often related to childhood abuse
   - Overlearned, maladaptive habit
   - Pleasure seeking and pain avoidance
   - Family traits, including lack of stability, lack of positive role models, lack of trust, inability to treat children as individuals, and parental addiction
3. *Sociocultural factors*
   - Availability and social acceptability of drug use
   - Societal ambivalence about or use or abuse of various substances, such as tobacco, alcohol, and marijuana
   - Cultural attitudes, values, norms, and sanctions
   - Nationality, ethnicity, and religion
   - Poverty with associated family instability and limited opportunities

Precipitating Stressors

Withdrawal

Table 17-2 presents general behaviors related to withdrawal from substances.

NURSE ALERT.   A serious and potentially life-threatening alcohol withdrawal disorder is *alcohol withdrawal delirium,* formerly known as *delirium tremens* (DTs). It usually occurs on the second or third day after the last drink has been taken and ends 48 to 72 hours after onset. Behaviors include the following:

1. Tremor
2. Anxiety
3. Paranoid delusions
4. Visual hallucinations
5. Disorientation
6. Elevated temperature
7. Tachycardia
8. Tachypnea
9. Hyperpnea
10. Vomiting
11. Diarrhea
12. Diaphoresis

Another serious behavioral manifestation that may result from alcohol withdrawal is grand mal convulsions. These do not usually recur once alcohol withdrawal is completed.

A person can predict the severity and duration of withdrawal symptoms by using the following three rules of thumb:

1. The longer the time between last use and appearance of withdrawal symptoms, and the longer these symptoms last, the less intense they will be.
2. The longer the half-life of the drug, the longer withdrawal symptoms will last.
3. The longer the half-life of the drug, the less intense the withdrawal symptoms will be.

NURSE ALERT.   Substance use during pregnancy can result in the development of fetal alcohol syndrome or the birth of an addicted infant. Women should be encouraged to remain drug and alcohol free during pregnancy.

Appraisal of Stressor

The reasons why a person initiates use of substances may include curiosity, desire to be grown up, desire to rebel against authority, peer pressure, desire to ease the pains of living, or desire to feel good. If the substance brings about the desired effects, use is likely to continue. As amount and frequency of substance use increase, so do the perceived stressors that provide a reason for more use. If substance use becomes associated with relief from emotional and social pain in the person's mind, the appraisal of these stressors will lead to more substance use. Perceiving the substance as the answer to these problems, the individual fails to develop healthier coping mechanisms. Gradually it takes more and more of the substance to achieve the same effect.

Coping Resources

Coping resources enable the person who abuses substances to survive and include the following:

- Effective communication and assertiveness skills
- Strong social support systems

- Alternative pleasurable activities
- Stress reduction techniques
- Vocational skills
- Motivation to change behavior

Coping Mechanisms

Substance abuse represents an unsuccessful attempt to cope. Healthier defense mechanisms and other adaptive behaviors are either inadequate or have not been developed. Ego defense mechanisms typically used by substance abusers include the following:

1. Denial of the problem
2. Rationalization
3. Projection of responsibility for the behavior
4. Minimization of the amount of alcohol or drug used

Nursing Diagnosis

The nurse should be aware that individuals who have substance abuse problems also tend to develop multiple physical problems, particularly if the substance abuse problem is severe. The complete plan of nursing care would include diagnosis of all the patient's nursing care needs. For the purposes of this discussion, nursing diagnoses are limited to those more specifically related to substance abuse. The box on p. 354 presents the primary and related NANDA nursing diagnoses for maladaptive chemically mediated responses.

Related Medical Diagnoses

Medical diagnoses related to maladaptive chemically mediated responses are based on the specific substance involved. The box on p. 355 describes these diagnoses.

Outcome Identification

The expected outcome for a patient with substance-related withdrawal follows:

The patient will overcome addiction safely and with a minimum of discomfort.

The expected outcome for a patient with substance-related dependence follows:

The patient will abstain from using all mood-altering chemicals.

NANDA Nursing Diagnoses Related to Maladaptive Chemically Mediated Responses

Anxiety
Communication, impaired verbal
*Coping, ineffective individual
*Family processes, altered: alcoholism
Grieving, dysfunctional
Growth and development, altered
Hopelessness
Infection, potential for
Injury, potential for
Knowledge deficit (specify)
Management of therapeutic regimen, individual or
    family: effective or ineffective
Noncompliance
Nutrition, altered
Parenting, altered
Powerlessness
Self-care deficit
Self-esteem disturbance
*Sensory/perceptual alterations
Sexual dysfunction
Sleep pattern disturbance
Social isolation
Spiritual distress
*Thought processes, altered
Violence, potential for

From North American Nursing Diagnosis Association: *NANDA nursing diagnoses: definitions and classification 1997-1998,* Philadelphia, 1997, The Association
*Primary nursing diagnosis for chemically mediated response.

DSM-IV Medical Diagnoses
Related to Maladaptive Chemically Mediated Responses

DSM-IV Diagnosis	Essential Features*
Substance dependence	Maladaptive pattern of substance use, characterized by any three of the following within 12 months: tolerance; withdrawal; using more of the substance or using for longer than planned; persistent desire but unsuccessful efforts to cut down or control use; much time spent in efforts to obtain, use, or recover from use; interference with social, occupational, or recreational activities; continued use despite knowledge of use-related recurrent physical or psychological problems.
Substance abuse	Maladaptive pattern of substance use, characterized by one or more of the following within 12 months: recurrent use resulting in failure to meet role obligations, recurrent use in physically hazardous situations, recurrent use-related legal problems, continued use despite persistent or recurrent use-related social or interpersonal problems. Has never met the criteria for dependence for the class of substance.

Modified from American Psychiatric Association: *Diagnostic and statistical manual of mental disorders*, ed 4 (DSM-IV), Washington, DC, 1994, The Association.

*A single set of essential features has been developed for substance dependence and for substance abuse. The essential features of intoxication and withdrawal vary according to the substance and are listed in Table 17-2.

Planning

A Patient Education Plan for prevention of substance abuse is presented on p. 357.

Implementation

> **NURSE ALERT.** Withdrawal from dependence on alcohol or drugs may result in life-threatening physical symptoms. The nurse should be familiar with the withdrawal symptoms presented in Table 17-2 and provide appropriate supportive interventions. Any unexpected behaviors or unanticipated worsening of the patient's condition should be reported to the physician promptly.

> **NURSE ALERT.** Unanticipated serious physiological distress in a patient who is a known or suspected substance abuser may be a sign of overdose. The nurse should be familiar with the behaviors associated with overdose of frequently abused substances, as described in Table 17-2. If overdose is suspected, the physician should be notified immediately.

Biological Interventions

Intervening in withdrawal

Substances with potentially life-threatening courses of withdrawal include alcohol, barbiturates, and benzodiazepines. Withdrawal from opiates and stimulants can be extremely uncomfortable but is generally not dangerous, although a patient may become suicidal during the acute phase of cocaine withdrawal. Withdrawal from the general depressants, opiates, and stimulants is treated by gradual tapering of a drug in the same classification and treatment with symptom-specific medication. No identified acute withdrawal pattern is associated with marijuana, hallucinogens, or PCP.

Patient Education Plan
Preventing Substance Abuse

Content	Instructional Activities	Evaluation
Elicit perceptions of substance use.	Lead group discussion about chemical use and experience with it. Correct misperceptions.	Patient describes accurate information about substance use.
Demonstrate negative effects of substance abuse.	Show films of physical and psychological effects of substance abuse. Provide written materials.	Patient identifies and describes physical and psychological effects of substance abuse.
Provide interaction with peer who has abused chemicals.	Initiate small group discussion with peer group member who has abused substances and quit because of negative experiences.	Patient compares and contrasts advantages and disadvantages of using mind-altering substances.
Obtain agreement to abstain from use of mind-altering substances.	Discuss future plans for refusing abused chemicals if offered.	Patient verbally agrees to abstain from using mind-altering substances.

Intervening in toxic psychosis

Acute toxic psychosis may result from ingestion of hallucinogens or PCP. Hallucinogen users need interpersonal intervention with constant reassurance. PCP users respond poorly to interpersonal stimulation and need to be kept in a quiet, protected environment. These patients may be terrified by the disturbances in perception that result from use of these drugs. They may act impulsively out of fear and harm themselves. Adequate staff should be available to manage this impulse behavior.

Intervening to maintain abstinence

Maintaining abstinence from abused substances is one of the most difficult issues in working with patients who have substance-related disorders. In treatment for addictions, mild levels of anxiety and depression can generate motivation for change. Therefore these symptoms should not be treated with medication unless they significantly interfere with the patient's functioning and participation in the treatment plan. However, a number of pharmacological therapies can help patients decrease cravings and maintain abstinence: (1) disulfiram (Antabuse), (2) naltrexone (Trexan), (3) opiate agonists, including methadone and LAAM, and (4) Acamprosate.

NURSE ALERT. Disulfiram (Antabuse) sensitizes alcoholic patients to alcohol. Ingestion of alcohol while taking Antabuse can lead to serious physical symptoms, possibly resulting in death. Symptoms include severe headache, nausea and vomiting, flushing, hypotension, tachycardia, dyspnea, diaphoresis, chest pain, palpitations, dizziness, and confusion. It can also lead to respiratory and cardiac collapse, unconsciousness, convulsions, and death.

The patient must be educated about the potential consequences of drinking while taking this drug. Patient education should also include the provision of a written list of alcohol-containing preparations to be avoided, including cough medicines, rubbing compounds, vinegars, aftershave lotions, and some mouthwashes. Drinking must be avoided for 14 days after disulfiram has been taken.

NURSE ALERT.   Naltrexone is the first drug approved by the U.S. Food and Drug Administration (FDA) for the treatment of alcohol dependence in more than 40 years. It blocks the euphoric effects of alcohol in the brain and promises new hope for substance abusers.

NURSE ALERT.   Acamprosate is the newest drug to help prevent relapse in alcoholism. It has no sedative, antianxiety, muscle relaxant, or antidepressant properties and produces no withdrawal symptoms. Acamprosate appears to work by lowering the activity of receptors for the excitatory neurotransmitter glutamate.

Interpersonal and Social System Interventions

Approaches to the substance abuser should include efforts to engage the patient interpersonally and to assist the person to find non-drug-using social supports in the community. Family counseling and self-help groups such as Alcoholics Anonymous (AA) may be particularly helpful.

Nursing interventions with the substance-abusing patient are summarized in the Nursing Treatment Plan Summary on pp. 362-365.

Interventions with Dually Diagnosed Patients

The dually diagnosed patient needs treatment for both disorders. The best treatment is an integrated one that combines pharmacological, psychosocial, and supportive services. Since both mental illness and substance abuse are chronic, relapsing conditions, the course of treatment can be expected to take considerable time. Table 17-3 describes stages of treatment and related goals and interventions for working with the dually diagnosed patient.

NURSE ALERT.   Since most abused drugs cross the placental barrier, women should be counseled about the possible effects of substance use during pregnancy. The safest

Table 17-3   Treatment stages, goals, and interventions for dually diagnosed patients

Treatment Stage	Suggested Goals and Interventions
Engagement	*Goal:* Development of working relationship between patient and nurse
	Interventions: Intervene in crises; assist with practical living problems; establish rapport with family members; demonstrate caring and support; listen actively.
Persuasion	*Goal:* Patient acceptance of having a substance abuse problem and the need for active change strategies
	Interventions: Help to analyze pros and cons of substance use; educate patient and family; arrange peer group discussions: expose patient to "double-trouble" self-help groups; adjust medication; persuade patient of need to comply with medication regimen.
Active treatment	*Goal:* Abstinence from substance use and compliance with medication regimen
	Interventions: Assist to change thinking patterns, friends, habits, behaviors, and living situations as necessary to support goals; teach social skills; encourage to develop positive social supports through double-trouble self-help groups; enlist family support of changes; monitor urine and breath for substances; offer disulfiram (Antabuse).
Relapse prevention	*Goal:* Absence or minimization of return to substance abuse
	Interventions: Reinforce abstinence, compliance, and behavioral changes; identify risk factors and help to practice preventive strategies; encourage continued involvement in double-trouble groups; continued laboratory monitoring.

pregnancy is one in which the mother is totally drug and alcohol free, with one exception: for pregnant women addicted to heroin, methadone maintenance is safer for the fetus than acute opiate detoxification.

Evaluation

The evaluation of substance abuse treatment is based on accomplishment of the expected outcomes and short-term goals. Estes, Smith-DiJulio, and Heinemann[1] have identified the following evaluation criteria for the treatment of alcoholic patients, which apply to abusers of other drugs as well:

1. Has the patient been able to progress significantly toward achieving the stated goals?
2. Can the patient usually communicate without being defensive?
3. Is the patient able to react appropriately, managing the demands of daily life without use of a drug?
4. Is the patient actively involved in a variety of activities, using external social and activity resources?
5. Does the patient use internal resources to be consistently productive at work and involved in meaningful interpersonal relationships?

Nursing Treatment Plan Summary
Maladaptive Chemically Mediated Responses

Nursing Diagnosis: Ineffective individual coping
Expected Outcome: Patient will abstain from using all mood-altering chemicals.

Short-term Goals	Interventions	Rationale
Patient will substitute healthy coping responses for substance-abusing behavior.	Confront patient with substance-abusing behavior and its consequences.	Motivation for change is related to recognition of a problem that is upsetting to the individual.
	Assist patient to identify substance abuse problem.	Identification of predisposing factors and precipitating stressors must precede planning for more adaptive behavioral responses.
	Involve patient in describing situations that lead to substance-abusing behavior.	
	Consistently offer support and the expectation that patient does have the strength to overcome the problem.	
Patient will assume responsibility for behavior.	Encourage patient to agree to participate in a treatment program.	Denial and rationalization are dysfunctional coping mechanisms that can interfere with recovery.
	Develop with patient a written contract for behavioral change that is signed by patient and nurse.	Personal commitment will enhance the likelihood of successful abstinence.
	Assist patient to identify and adopt healthier coping responses.	

Patient will identify and use social support systems.	Identify and assess social support systems available to patient.	Substance abusers are often dependent and socially isolated people who use drugs to gain confidence in social situations.
	Provide support to significant others.	Substance-abusing behavior alienates significant others, thus increasing the person's isolation.
	Educate patient and significant others about the substance abuse problem and available resources.	It is difficult to manipulate people who have participated in the same behaviors.
	Refer patient to appropriate resources and provide support until patient is involved in the program.	Social support systems must be readily available over time and acceptable to patient.

Continued

Nursing Treatment Plan Summary
Maladaptive Chemically Mediated Responses—cont'd

Nursing Diagnosis: Altered thought processes
Expected Outcome: Patient will overcome addiction safely and with a minimum of discomfort.

Short-term Goals	Interventions	Rationale
Patient will withdraw from dependence on the abused substance.	Provide supportive physical care: vital signs, nutrition, hydration, seizure precautions. Administer medication according to detoxification schedule.	Detoxification of the physically dependent person can be dangerous and is always uncomfortable. Patient's physical safety must receive high priority for nursing intervention.
Patient will be oriented to time, place, person, and situation.	Assess orientation frequently; orient patient if needed; place a clock and calendar where patient can see them.	Cognitive function is usually affected by addiction; disorientation is frightening.

Patient will report symptoms of withdrawal.	Observe carefully for withdrawal symptoms and report suspected withdrawal immediately.	Withdrawal symptoms provide powerful motivation for continued substance abuse; judgment may be impaired by substance use.
Patient will correctly interpret environmental stimuli.	Explain all nursing interventions; assign consistent staff; keep soft light on in room; avoid loud noises; encourage trusted family and friends to stay with patient.	Sensory and perceptual alterations related to use of drugs or alcohol are frightening; consistency reduces need to interpret stimuli.
Patient will recognize and talk about hallucinations or delusions.	Observe for response to internal stimuli; encourage patient to describe hallucinations or delusions; explain relationship of these experiences to withdrawal from addictive substances.	Assisting patient to identify delusional or hallucinatory experiences and relate them to withdrawal is reassuring.

your **INTERNET**
c o n n e c t i o n

Dual Diagnosis Website
http://www.erols.com/ksciacca/
WEB of Addictions
http://www.well.com/user/woa/

Reference

1. Estes NJ, Smith-DiJulio K, Heinemann ME: *Nursing diagnosis of the alcoholic person,* St Louis, 1982, Mosby.

Suggested readings

American Nurses' Association and National Nurses Society on Addictions: *Standards of addictions nursing practice with selected diagnoses and criteria,* Kansas City, Mo, 1988, The Association.

American Psychiatric Association: Practice guideline for the treatment of patients with substance use disorders: alcohol, cocaine, opioids, *Am J Psychiatry* 152:11, 1995.

American Psychiatric Association: Practice guideline for the treatment of patients with nicotine dependence, *Am J Psychiatry* 153(suppl):1, 1996.

Bachmann K et al: An integrated treatment program for dually diagnosed patients, *Psychiatric Serv* 3:314, 1997.

Boyd M, Hauenstein E: Psychiatric assessment and confirmation of dual disorders in rural substance abusing women, *Arch Psychiatric Nurs* 2:74, 1997.

Carey K: Treatment of co-occurring substance abuse and major mental illness, *New Dir Ment Health Serv* 70:19, 1996.

Finke L, Williams J, Stanley R: Nurses referred to a peer assistance program for alcohol and drug problems, *Arch Psychiatr Nurs* 10:319, 1996.

Humphreys K, Moos R, Cohen C: Social and community resources and long-term recovery from treated and untreated alcoholism, *J Stud Alcohol* 5:231, 1997.

Jerrell J: Toward cost-effective care for persons with dual diagnoses, *J Ment Health Admin* 23:329, 1996.

Miele G, Trautman K, Hasin D: Assessing comorbid mental and substance-use disorders: a guide for clinical practice, *J Pract Psychiatry Behav Health* 2:272, 1996.

Mynatt S: A model of contributing risk factors to chemical dependency in nurses, *J Psychosoc Nurs* 34:13, 1996.

Stuart G, Laraia M: *Principles and practice of psychiatric nursing,* ed 6, St Louis, 1998, Mosby.

Eating Regulation Responses and Eating Disorders

18

Continuum of Eating Regulation Responses

As a pattern of self-regulation, properly controlled eating contributes to psychological, biological, and sociocultural health and well-being. Adaptive eating responses are characterized by balanced eating patterns, appropriate caloric intake, and body weight that is appropriate for height and frame. Illnesses associated with maladaptive eating regulation responses include anorexia nervosa, bulimia nervosa, and binge eating disorder (Fig. 18-1). These disorders can cause biological changes, including altered metabolic rates, profound malnutrition, and possibly death.

Prevalence

Anorexia nervosa

Anorexia nervosa occurs in about 1% to 2% of the female population, with onset often between ages 13 and 20. An estimated one in 10 people with anorexia is male.

Bulimia nervosa

Bulimia is more common than anorexia, with estimates of 2% to 3% of the female population and a prevalence of 4% to 15% of

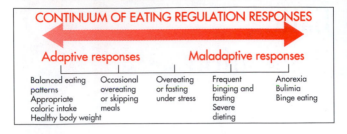

Figure 18-1
Continuum of eating regulation responses.

female high-school and college students. The age of onset is typically ages 15 to 18. An estimated one in five people with bulimia is male.

Assessment

Patients with maladaptive eating regulation responses must receive a comprehensive nursing assessment, including complete biological, psychological, and sociocultural evaluation. A full physical examination should be performed, with particular attention to vital signs, weight for height, skin, the cardiovascular system, and evidence of laxative or diuretic abuse and vomiting. A dental examination may be indicated, and it is useful to assess growth, sexual development, and general physical development indicators. A psychiatric history, substance abuse history, and family assessment are also needed.

Behaviors

Box 18-1 lists key features of anorexia nervosa and bulimia nervosa.

Binge eating

Binge eating is the rapid consumption of large quantities of food in a discrete period, although no agreement exists on exactly how many calories constitute a binge. Emphasis on the individual's perception of loss of control and perceived excessive caloric intake is more important to the nursing assessment than the total number of calories consumed during a binge. Therefore

Box 18-1   Key Features of Anorexia Nervosa and Bulimia Nervosa

Anorexia Nervosa	Bulimia Nervosa
Rare vomiting or diuretic/laxative abuse	Frequent vomiting or diuretic/laxative abuse
More severe weight loss	Less weight loss
Slightly younger	Slightly older
More introverted	More extroverted
Hunger denied	Hunger experienced
Eating behavior may be considered normal and source of esteem	Eating behavior considered foreign and source of distress
Sexually inactive	More sexually active
Obsessional and perfectionistic features predominate	Avoidant, dependent, or borderline features as well as obsessional features
Death from starvation (or suicide in chronically ill patients)	Death from hypokalemia or suicide
Amenorrhea	Menses irregular or absent
More favorable prognosis	Less favorable prognosis
Fewer behavioral abnormalities (increase with severity)	Stealing, drug and alcohol abuse, self-mutilation, and other behavioral abnormalities

From Andersen AE: *Practical comprehensive treatment of anorexia nervosa and bulimia*, Baltimore, 1985, Johns-Hopkins University Press.

the nurse must carefully assess exactly what each person means by a binge.

Fasting or restricting

People with anorexia often do not consume more than 500 to 700 calories a day and may ingest as few as 200, but they consider their intake adequate for their energy needs. Some individuals with anorexia may not eat for days at a time. Despite these restrictions, many anorectic people are preoccupied or obsessed with food and may do much of the family cooking.

Purging

Individuals with eating disorders may use a variety of purging behaviors, including excessive exercise, over-the-counter and prescription diuretics, diet pills, laxatives, and steroids. Many patients engage in more than one purging behavior.

Medical and psychiatric complications

Almost every person with maladaptive eating regulation responses has some type of associated physical problem, because all body systems are affected. Many patients seeking treatment for eating disorders also have evidence of other psychiatric disorders, such as depression, obsessive-compulsive disorder, substance abuse disorders, and personality disorders.

Predisposing Factors

Biological

It is generally recognized that eating disorders are familial. First-degree female relatives of people with eating disorders are at higher risk than the general population. Concordance rates for eating disorders in monozygotic twins is 52% and in dizygotic twins 11%. A higher risk for other eating disorders and for depression also is seen in first-degree relatives of people with eating disorders, suggesting common etiological factors.

Biological models of the etiology of eating disorders focus on the appetite regulation center in the hypothalamus, which controls specific neurochemical mechanisms for feeding and satiety. Serotonin is thought to be involved in the pathophysiology of eating disorders, although these biological models are still in the developmental stage.

Environmental

A variety of environmental factors may predispose an individual to the development of an eating disorder. Early histories of patients with eating disorders are often complicated by medical and surgical illnesses, separations, family deaths, and conflicted family environments. Sexual abuse has been reported in 20% to 50% of patients with bulimia, but this rate may be similar to that found in patients with other psychiatric disorders.

Psychological

Most patients with eating disorders exhibit clusters of psychological symptoms, such as rigidity, ritualism, meticulousness, perfectionism, exactness, symmetry, greater risk avoidance and restraint, and poor impulse control. Early separation and individuation conflicts, a pervasive sense of ineffectiveness and helplessness, difficulty interpreting feelings and tolerating intense emotional states, and fear of biological or psychological maturity may predispose an individual to an eating disorder. Box 18-2 lists

---

Box 18-2   Psychological Characteristics Associated with Eating Disorders

Anxiety
Compulsivity
Conflict avoidance
Depression
Difficulty expressing feelings, particularly anger
Distorted self-image
Exaggerated sense of guilt
Fear of sexuality and biological maturity
Feelings of alienation
Intolerance for frustration
Low self-esteem
Obsession
Perfectionism
Poor impulse control
Self-consciousness
Sense of ineffectiveness

additional personality and psychological characteristics of these patients.

Sociocultural

In cultures where plumpness is either accepted or valued, eating disorders are rare. Also, the sociocultural environment for adolescents and young women in the United States places great emphasis on thinness and control over one's body as a yardstick for self-evaluation.

Precipitating Stressors

Individuals with the previous predisposing factors are especially vulnerable to environmental pressures or life stressors, such as the loss of a significant other, interpersonal rejection, and failure.

Appraisal of Stressor

In addition to a positive correlation existing between stress and the severity of eating disorders, the person's appraisal of the stress appears to play an important role, affecting both the treatment course and the treatment outcome.

Coping Resources

One of the most important aspects of the assessment of these patients is the level of their motivation to change their behavior. Patients may be asked to identify the advantages and disadvantages of giving up the behavior. This information can be used to evaluate a patient's insight, identify coping resources, and stimulate therapeutic issues for further discussion.

Coping Mechanisms

Anorectic patients most frequently use the defense mechanism of denial in a severely maladaptive way, and they usually do not seek help on their own. The defense mechanisms used by bulimic patients include avoidance, denial, isolation of affect, and intellectualization.

Nursing Diagnosis

The box on p. 373 presents the primary and related NANDA nursing diagnoses for maladaptive eating regulation responses. A

NANDA Nursing Diagnoses Related to Maladaptive Eating Regulation Responses

*Anxiety
*Body image disturbance
  Coping, ineffective individual
  Decisional conflict (specify)
  Denial, ineffective
  Family processes, altered
  Fatigue
*Fluid volume deficit
  Growth and development, altered
  Hopelessness
  Injury, risk for
  Loneliness, risk for
*Nutrition, altered
  Personal identity disturbance
*Powerlessness
  Role performance, altered
*Self-esteem disturbance
*Self-mutilation, risk for
  Sexual dysfunction
  Social interaction, impaired
*Therapeutic regimen: individual, ineffective management of
  Thought processes, altered

From North American Nursing Diagnosis Association: *NANDA nursing diagnoses: definitions and classification 1997-1998,* Philadelphia, 1997, The Association.
*Primary nursing diagnosis for eating problems.

complete nursing assessment would include all maladaptive responses of the patient. Additional nursing problems resulting from the eating disorder should also be identified.

Related Medical Diagnoses

The box on p. 374 identifies the medical diagnoses related to maladaptive eating regulation responses and their essential features.

DSM-IV Medical Diagnoses Related to Maladaptive Eating Regulation Responses

DSM-IV Diagnosis	Essential Features
Anorexia nervosa	Intense fear of gaining weight, even when underweight. A disturbance in the way the body is experienced and a refusal to maintain body weight above a minimal normal weight for age and height lead to a body weight 15% below expected. In females there is also the absence of at least three consecutive menstrual cycles.
Bulimia nervosa	Recurrent episodes of binge eating with a feeling of lack of control over the eating behavior and persistent overconcern with body shape and weight. The individual also regularly engages in self-induced vomiting, use of laxatives, or rigorous dieting and fasting to counteract the effects of binge eating.
Binge eating disorder	Recurrent episodes of binging that are a cause of distress with a feeling of lack of control over the eating behavior but without behaviors used to prevent weight gain.

Modified from American Psychiatric Association: *Diagnostic and statistical manual of mental disorders*, ed 4 (DSM-IV), Washington, DC, 1994, The Association.

Outcome Identification

The expected outcome for the patient with maladaptive eating regulation responses is:

The patient will restore healthy eating patterns and normalize physiological parameters related to body weight and nutrition.

Planning

Important considerations in the planning phase of the nursing process are the choice of an inpatient, outpatient, or partial hospitalization treatment setting and the formulation of a nurse-patient contract. Box 18-3 presents clinical criteria for hospitalizing a patient with an eating disorder. A Family Education Plan for preventing childhood eating problems is presented on pp. 376 and 377.

Box 18-3   Clinical Criteria for Hospitalization of Patients with an Eating Disorder

Medical

Need for extensive diagnostic evaluation
Weight loss greater than 30% of body weight over
    3 months
Heart rate less than 40 beats per minute
Temperature less than 36° C or 96.8° F
Systolic blood pressure less than 70 mm Hg
Serum potassium less than 2.5 mEq/L despite oral potas-
    sium replacement
Severe dehydration
Concurrent somatic illnesses (e.g., infection)

Psychiatric

Risk of suicide or self-mutilation
Severe depression
Psychosis
Inadequate response to outpatient treatment

Family Education Plan
Preventing Childhood Eating Problems

Content	Instructional Activities	Evaluation
Describe self-demand feeding and its importance in healthy eating behaviors.	Explore current feeding practices of parents and understanding of healthy eating. Provide information to enhance knowledge of healthy eating behaviors.	Parents identify healthy eating behaviors and self-demand feeding and begin to explore how their relationship with food influences their children's eating.
Describe physiological and psychological signs of hunger and satiety, as well as the meaning of and differences between both types. Describe danger of psychological hunger.	Explore parents' own signs of hunger and satiety and also have parents describe their children's signs. Explain the use of a hunger diary, which is a daily journal regarding signs of hunger.	Parents keep a hunger diary to record physical and psychological signs of hunger and satiety for themselves and their children. Parents can distinguish between psychological and physical hunger.

Explore myths about feeding, e.g., "cleaning the plate" and "eating because other children are starving."	Describe the importance of allowing children to determine their feeding needs and the relationship of healthy eating to childrens' ability to differentiate between physical and psychological signs of hunger and satiety. Give homework assignment for each parent to interview three other adults about their current eating practices and memories of eating.	Parents complete homework assignment, discuss interview experiences, and describe how perpetuating myths about feeding can harm their children.
Implement self-demand feeding at particular developmental stages of children.	Review the stages that children experience with eating and the potential problems they may have at each stage.	Parents discuss the developmental stages of their children and plan for implementing self-demand feeding.
Discuss parental experiences related to implementing self-demand feeding.	Review parents' expectations and experiences with implementing self-demand feeding.	Parents relate any problem with self-demand feeding. Nurse evaluates family for further education and plans for follow-up if necessary.

Implementation

The nursing care for a patient with an eating disorder includes the following areas of intervention:
1. Nutritional stabilization
2. Exercise monitoring
3. Cognitive behavioral interventions
4. Body image interventions
5. Family involvement
6. Group therapies
7. Medication

A Nursing Treatment Plan Summary for patients with maladaptive eating regulation responses is presented on pp. 379-382.

Evaluation

1. Have normal eating patterns been restored?
2. Have the biological and psychological sequelae of malnutrition been corrected?
3. Have the associated sociocultural and behavioral problems been resolved so that relapse does not occur?

Nursing Treatment Plan Summary
Maladaptive Eating Regulation Responses

Nursing Diagnosis: Altered nutrition
Expected Outcome: Patient will restore healthy eating patterns and normalize physiological parameters related to body weight and nutrition.

Short-term Goals	Interventions	Rationale
Patient will engage in treatment and acknowledge having an eating disorder.	Help patient identify maladaptive eating responses.	First step of treatment is for patient to acknowledge the illness and see the need for help.
	Discuss positive and negative consequences of maladaptive eating responses.	
	Contract with patient to engage in treatment.	
Patient will be able to describe a balanced diet based on the five food groups.	Complete a nutritional assessment, including eating-related behaviors and preferences.	Knowledge of healthy nutrition is essential to establishing and maintaining adaptive eating responses.
	Teach, clarify, and reinforce knowledge of proper nutrition.	

Continued

Nursing Treatment Plan Summary
Maladaptive Eating Regulation Responses—cont'd

Short-term Goals	Interventions	Rationale
Patient's nutritional status will be stabilized by a specified target date.	Monitor physiological status for signs of compromised nutrition. Administer medications and somatic treatments for management of symptoms. Monitor and evaluate patient's response to somatic treatments. Implement nursing activities as specified in the program contract and protocol.	Weight stabilization must be a central and early goal for the nutritionally compromised patient. Medications may assist the appetite regulation center and neurochemical responses to feeding and satiety.
Patient will participate daily in a balanced exercise program.	Review established exercise routines. Modify exercise patterns, focusing on physical fitness rather than weight reduction. Reinforce new exercise and fitness behaviors.	Focus of a balanced exercise program should be on physical fitness rather than calorie reduction to lose weight.

Nursing Diagnosis: Body image disturbance

Expected Outcome: Patient will express clear and accurate descriptions of body size, body boundaries, and ideal weight.

Patient will correct body image distortions.	Modify body image misperceptions through cognitive and behavioral strategies. Use dance and movement therapies to enhance the integration of mind and body. Employ imagery and relaxation interventions to decrease anxiety related to body perceptions.	Body image distortions involve perceptions, attitudes, and behaviors that place so much emphasis on appearance that they define self-worth.
Patient will modify cognitive distortions about body weight, shape, and eating responses.	Assist patient in identifying: 1. Cues that trigger problematic eating responses and body image concerns 2. Thoughts, feelings, and assumptions associated with the specific cues 3. Connections between these thoughts, feelings, and assumptions and eating regulation responses 4. Consequences resulting from the eating responses	Cognitive distortions result in lowered self-esteem. Behavioral change occurs as a result of increased awareness of feelings and faulty cognitions.

Continued

Nursing Treatment Plan Summary
Maladaptive Eating Regulation Responses—cont'd

Short-term Goals	Interventions	Rationale
Patient will identify social support systems that reinforce accurate body perceptions and adaptive eating responses.	Include family members in the evaluation and treatment planning process. Assess family as a system and impact of the eating disorder on family functioning. Initiate group therapy to mobilize social support and reinforce adaptive responses.	Patients with eating disorders benefit from involvement of family members and supportive group work.

your **INTERNET**
c o n n e c t i o n

Anorexia Nervosa and Bulimia Association
http://qlink.queensu.ca/~4map/anabhome.htm
The Something Fishy Website on Eating Disorders
http://www.something-fishy.com/ed.htm

Suggested readings

American Psychiatric Association: Practice guidelines: practice guidelines for eating disorders, *Am J Psychiatry* 150:207, 1993.

Brewerton TD: Toward a unified theory of serotonin dysregulation in eating and related disorders, *Psychoneuroendocrinology* 20:6, 1995.

Garner D, Garfinkel P: *Handbook of treatment for eating disorders,* New York, 1997, Guilford Publications.

Harper-Giuffre H, MacKenzie K: *Group psychotherapy for eating disorders,* Washington DC, 1992, American Psychiatric Press.

Hirschmann J, Zaphiropoulos L: *Preventing childhood eating problems: a practical positive approach to raising children free of food and weight conflicts,* Carlsbad CA, 1993, Gurze Books.

Irwin E: A focused overview of anorexia nervosa and bulimia: Part I. Etiological Issues; Part II. Challenges to the practice of psychiatric nursing, *Arch Psych Nurs* 7:342, 1993.

Kaplan A, Garfinkel P, eds: *Medical issues and the eating disorders,* New York, 1993, Brunner/Mazel.

McGowan A, Whitbread J: Out of control! The most effective way to help the binge-eating patient, *J Psychosoc Nurs* 34:30, 1996.

Owen SV, Fullerton ML: Would it make a difference? A discussion group in a behaviorally oriented inpatient eating disorder program, *J Psychosoc Nurs* 33:35, 1995.

Stein K: The self-schema model: a theoretical approach to the self-concept in eating disorders, *Arch Psych Nurs* 2:96, 1996.

Stuart G, Laraia M: *Principles and practice of psychiatric nursing,* ed 6, St Louis, 1998, Mosby.

Sullivan PF: Mortality in anorexia nervosa, *Am J Psychiatry* 152:7, 1995.

Wiederman MW, Pryor TL: Overcoming anorexia nervosa, *J Pract Psychiatry Behav Health* 2:5, 1996.

Wolfe BE: Dimensions of response to antidepressant agents in bulimia nervosa: a review, *Arch Psychiatr Nurs* 3:111, 1995.

Zerbe K: *The body betrayed: women, eating disorders, and treatment,* Washington DC, 1993, American Psychiatric Association Press.

Sexual Responses and Sexual Disorders

19

Continuum of Sexual Responses

Sexuality is broadly defined as a desire for contact, warmth, tenderness, or love. It includes looking and talking, handholding, kissing, or self-pleasuring; and the production of mutual orgasm. Sexuality is a part of a person's total sense of self.

Experts in the area of sexuality do not agree on what types of sexual behaviors are "normal." Expressions of sexuality can be viewed on a continuum ranging from adaptive to maladaptive (Fig. 19-1). The most adaptive sexual responses are seen as behaviors that meet the following criteria:

1. Between two consenting adults
2. Mutually satisfying to the individuals involved
3. Not psychologically or physically harmful to either party
4. Lacking in force or coercion
5. Conducted in private

Maladaptive sexual responses include behaviors that do not meet one or more of these criteria.

Caution must be used when attempting to label sexual behaviors as adaptive or maladaptive. For instance, sexual behavior can meet the criteria but still be unsatisfactory for an individual if altered by the impact of what society dictates as acceptable and unacceptable behavior.

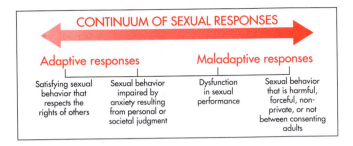

Figure 19-1
Continuum of sexual responses.

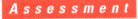

Self-Awareness of the Nurse

The most critical element in being able to counsel patients competently about sexuality is nurses' awareness of their own feelings and values. Nurses' level of self-awareness has a direct impact on their ability to intervene effectively with patients.

Behaviors

Many modes of sexual expression exists. In 1948 Kinsey used a seven-point rating scale in examining sexual preference (Fig. 19-2) in which 0 represented exclusively heterosexual experiences, 6 represented exclusively homosexual experiences, and 2, 3, or 4 indicated bisexuality. He suggested that most individuals are not exclusively heterosexual or homosexual. The following are definitions of common terms:

1. *Heterosexual*—a person who is sexually attracted to members of the opposite sex
2. *Homosexual*—a person who is sexually attracted to members of the same sex
3. *Bisexual*—a person who is sexually attracted to people of both sexes
4. *Transvestite*—a person who dresses in the clothes of the opposite sex
5. *Transsexual*—a person who is genetically an anatomical male or female, but who expresses, with strong conviction, that he or she has the mind of the opposite sex, and seeks to

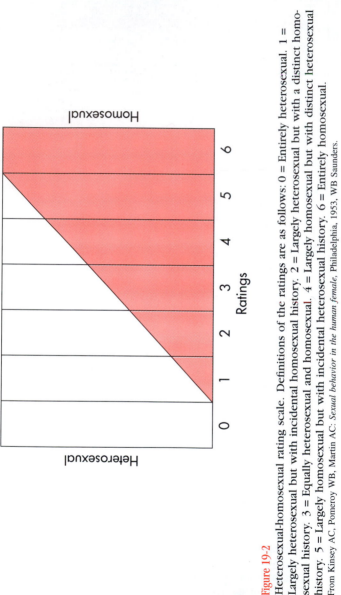

Figure 19-2

Heterosexual-homosexual rating scale. Definitions of the ratings are as follows: 0 = Entirely heterosexual. 1 = Largely heterosexual but with incidental homosexual history. 2 = Largely heterosexual but with a distinct homosexual history. 3 = Equally heterosexual and homosexual. 4 = Largely homosexual but with distinct heterosexual history. 5 = Largely homosexual but with incidental heterosexual history. 6 = Entirely homosexual.

From Kinsey AC, Pomeroy WB, Martin AC: *Sexual behavior in the human female*, Philadelphia, 1953, WB Saunders.

change his or her sex legally and through hormonal and surgical sex reassignment

Predisposing Factors

At present, no one theory can adequately explain the process of sexual development or the factors predisposing a person to maladaptive sexual responses. Several theories have been postulated, as follows:

1. *Biological factors.* These are initially responsible for the development of gender, that is, whether a person is genetically male or female. The person's somatotype includes chromosomes, hormones, internal and external genitalia, and gonads.

2. *Psychoanalytical view.* Freud viewed sexuality as one of the key forces of human life. He was the first theorist to believe that sexuality was developed before the onset of puberty and that a person's choice of sexual expression depended on an interplay of heredity, biology, and social factors. He proposed that the development of sexuality was specifically related to the development of object relations during the psychosocial stages of development.

3. *Behavioral view.* This perspective views sexual behavior as a measurable response with both physiological and psychological components to a learned stimulus or reinforcement event. The treatment of sexual problems involves processes to change behavior through direct intervention without the need to identify underlying causes or psychodynamics.

Precipitating Stressors

Sexual identity cannot be separated from a person's self-concept or body image. Therefore, when changes occur in the person's body or emotions, sexual responses change as well. Specific threats include the following:

1. Physical illness and injury
2. Psychiatric illness
3. Medications
4. Human immunodeficiency virus (HIV), acquired immunodeficiency syndrome (AIDS)
5. The aging process

Appraisal of Stressor

Feelings about oneself as a sexual being change throughout the life cycle and are greatly influenced by a person's appraisal of the stressful situation.

Coping Resources

Coping resources may include the individual's knowledge about sexuality, positive sexual experiences in the past, supportive individuals including the person's sexual partner, and social or cultural norms that encourage healthy expression.

Coping Mechanisms

Numerous coping mechanisms may be used in the expression of a person's sexual response, including the following:

1. *Fantasy* may be used to enhance sexual experiences.
2. *Denial* may be used to refuse to recognize sexual conflicts or dissatisfactions.
3. *Rationalization* may be used to justify or make acceptable otherwise unacceptable sexual impulses, feelings, behaviors, or motives.
4. *Withdrawal* may be used to cope with unresolved feelings about becoming vulnerable and with the resulting ambivalent feelings about intimacy.

Nursing Diagnosis

The primary NANDA nursing diagnoses are altered sexuality patterns, which include lack of sexual satisfaction and conflicts involving sex roles and values, and sexual dysfunction, which includes actual physical limitations. The box on p. 389 presents the primary and related NANDA diagnoses for variations in sexual response.

Related Medical Diagnoses

Many people who experience transient variations in sexual response have no medically diagnosed health problem. Patients with more severe or persistent problems are classified in one of three basic categories of DSM-IV: gender identity disorders, paraphilias, and sexual dysfunctions. The box on pp. 390 and 391 describes the specific medical diagnoses in each of these diagnostic classes.

NANDA Nursing Diagnoses Related to Variations in Sexual Response

Anxiety
Body image disturbance
Decisional conflict
Fear
Grieving, dysfunctional
Health maintenance, altered
Health-seeking behaviors (specify)
Loneliness, risk for
Pain
Personal identity disturbance
Powerlessness
Role performance, altered
Self-care deficit (specify)
Self-esteem disturbance
Sensory/perceptual alterations (specify)
*Sexual dysfunction
*Sexuality patterns, altered
Social interaction, impaired
Spiritual distress

From North American Nursing Diagnosis Association: *NANDA nursing diagnoses: definitions and classification 1997-1998,* Philadelphia, 1997, The Association.
*Primary nursing diagnosis for variations in sexual response.

Outcome Identification

The expected outcome for patients with maladaptive sexual responses is:

The patient will obtain the maximum level of adaptive sexual responses to enhance or maintain health.

Planning

Education is the usual method of primary prevention for sexual problems and issues. A Patient Education Plan for teaching about sexual response after an organic illness is presented on p. 392.

DSM-IV Medical Diagnoses Related to Variations in Sexual Response

DSM-IV Diagnosis	Essential Features
Hypoactive sexual disorder	Persistent or recurrent deficit or absence of sexual fantasies and desire for sexual activity.
Sexual aversion disorder	Persistent or recurrent extreme aversion to and avoidance of all or almost all genital sexual contact with a sexual partner.
Sexual arousal disorder	Persistent or recurrent partial or complete failure to attain or maintain the physiological response of sexual activity, or persistent or recurrent lack of a subjective sense of sexual excitement and pleasure during sexual activity.
Orgasmic disorder	Persistent or recurrent delay in or absence of orgasm after a normal sexual excitement phase during sexual activity that the clinician judges to be adequate in focus, intensity, and duration, taking into account the individual's age.
Premature ejaculation	Persistent or recurrent ejaculation with minimal sexual stimulation, before, during, or shortly after penetration, before the individual desires it.
Dyspareunia	Recurrent or persistent genital pain before, during, or after sexual intercourse.
Vaginismus	Recurrent or persistent involuntary spasm of the musculature of the outer third of the vagina that interferes with coitus.
Sexual dysfunction due to a general medical condition	Clinically significant sexual dysfunction etiologically related to a general medical condition.
Substance-induced sexual dysfunction	Clinically significant sexual dysfunction that developed during significant substance intoxication or withdrawal.

Exhibitionism	Persistent association, lasting at least 6 months, between intense sexual arousal, desire, acts, or fantasies and exposing one's genitals to an unsuspecting stranger.
Fetishism	Persistent association, lasting at least 6 months, between intense sexual arousal, desire, acts, or fantasies and nonliving objects (e.g., female undergarments).
Frotteurism	Persistent association, lasting at least 6 months, between intense sexual arousal, desire, acts, or fantasies and rubbing against a nonconsenting person.
Pedophilia	Persistent association, lasting at least 6 months, between intense sexual arousal, desire, acts, or fantasies and one or more children, aged 13 years or younger.
Sexual masochism	Persistent association, lasting at least 6 months, between intense sexual arousal, desire, acts, or fantasies and being humiliated, beaten, bound, or otherwise being made to suffer (real or imagined).
Sexual sadism	Persistent association, lasting at least 6 months, between intense sexual arousal, desire, acts, or fantasies and the affliction of real or simulated psychological or physical suffering (including humiliation).
Voyeurism	Persistent association, lasting at least 6 months, between intense sexual arousal, desire, acts, or fantasies and observing unsuspecting people who are naked, in the act of disrobing, or engaging in sexual activity.
Transvestic fetishism	Persistent association, lasting at least 6 months, between intense sexual arousal, desire, acts, or fantasies and cross-dressing.
Gender identity disorder of childhood, adolescence, or adulthood	Persistent and intense distress about being a male or a female, with an intense desire to be the opposite sex, a preoccupation of adulthood with the activities of the opposite sex, and a repudiation of one's own anatomical structures.

Modified from American Psychiatric Association: *Diagnostic and statistical manual of mental disorders*, ed 4 (DSM-IV), Washington, DC, 1994, The Association.

Patient Education Plan
Sexual Response After an Organic Illness

Content	Instructional Activities	Evaluation
Describe the variety of human sexual response patterns.	Discuss range of sexual desires, modes of expression, and techniques.	Patient identifies preferences and typical level of sexual functioning.
Define patient's primary organic problem.	Provide accurate information on disruption caused by the organic impairment.	Patient understands nature of the organic illness.
Clarify relationship between patient's organic problem and level of sexual functioning.	Reframe distorted or confused perceptions about impact of illness on sexual functioning.	Patient accurately describes the impact of illness on sexual functioning.
Identify ways to enhance patient's sexual functioning and improve interpersonal communication.	Describe additional experiences that would enhance sexual satisfaction and the relationship between patient and partner.	Patient and partner report reduced anxiety and greater satisfaction with sexual responses.

Implementation

Intervening in Health Education

Before engaging in either health education or counseling, nurses must examine their own values and beliefs about patients who practice sexual behavior that may be different. This can be facilitated by exploring typical myths about human sexuality held by society (Table 19-1).

Intervening in Sexual Responses in the Nurse-Patient Relationship

Feelings of sexual attraction and sexual fantasies are part of the human experience, and the nurse should address them. Two aspects of this include a nurse's sexual attraction to a patient and the patient's sexual acting out or display of seductive behaviors toward the nurse. Table 19-2 summarizes considerations in sexual responses of patients to nurses.

Patients may also experience maladaptive sexual responses resulting from physical and emotional illness, sexual preference, gender identity, or dysfunctions of the sexual response cycle. A Nursing Treatment Plan Summary for maladaptive sexual responses is presented on pp. 399-401.

Evaluation

1. Were the nurse's own feelings and values about sexuality explored and handled appropriately in giving patient care?
2. Was the nursing assessment of the patient's sexuality complete, accurate, and done professionally?
3. Have the patient's feelings about self improved during treatment?
4. If the patient was dysfunctional, was functional ability improved or restored?
5. Was health teaching on variations in sexual expression appropriately carried out?
6. Have the patient's interpersonal relationships improved?
7. Did the patient think that the care was helpful in meeting health-care goals?
8. Is referral to another health-care professional or agency indicated for the patient?

Table 19-1 Ten common myths and facts about human sexuality

Myth	Result of Myth	Fact
Patients become embarrassed when nurses bring up the subject of sexuality and would prefer that nurses not ask questions about sex.	If nurses believe this, they deny patients the opportunity to ask questions and clarify concerns related to sexual issues.	Patients would prefer that nurses initiate discussions of sexuality with them.
Excessive masturbation is harmful.	Individuals often feel guilty or ashamed about masturbating; some deny themselves this experience because of uncomfortable feelings perpetuated by society.	No evidence indicates that masturbation causes physical problems. If masturbation leads to satisfaction and pleasure, it is unlikely to be a problem.
Sexual fantasies about having sex with a partner other than lover or spouse indicate relationship difficulties.	Individuals may become uncomfortable about having a fantasy with a different partner. They may experience guilt feelings and view the fantasy as a sign of infidelity.	Imagining sex with a different partner is a common sexual fantasy and does not necessarily indicate desire to act out the fantasized behavior.
Sex during menstruation is unclean and harmful.	Women often view their bodies as unclean and even unfit or inferior during menstruation. Women use menstruation as an excuse to avoid intercourse rather than simply saying no without a "good reason."	Medically, menstrual flow is not harmful or dirty. If women desire, no reason exists to abstain from intercourse during menstrual flow.

Oral and anal intercourse are perverted and dangerous.

Oral and anal intercourse are not harmful if certain precautions are taken when performing anal intercourse, such as avoiding vaginal contamination and wearing a condom to prevent disease transmission.

Many individuals refrain from these behaviors or indulge in them only to feel ashamed and guilty afterward.

Most homosexuals molest children.

Research shows that the adult heterosexual male poses a much greater risk to the underage child than the adult homosexual male.

Known homosexuals are often fired from teaching jobs, and many parents will not allow their children to spend time with any homosexual.

Homosexuals are sick and cannot control their sexual behavior.

Most homosexuals' social and psychological adjustment is the same as that of the heterosexual majority, and objectionable sexual advances are much more likely to be made by a heterosexual (usually male to female) than a homosexual.

Homosexuals are denied jobs and are sometimes jailed for their homosexuality. Homosexual partners may have their children taken away by courts.

Continued

Table 19-1 Ten common myths and facts about human sexuality—cont'd

Myth	Result of Myth	Fact
Because of sex education programs, most adolescents and young adults are aware of the risks of acquiring sexually transmitted diseases (STDs) and practice safe sex.	When health educators believe that young adults have adequate knowledge about STDs, they may not take the time to assess further, add to this knowledge, and correct any misconceptions.	A study of more than 500 freshmen at a large university reported that of those who had multiple partners, fewer than 50% used condoms to lower the risk of disease.
Advancing age means the end of sex.	Many older adults become victims of this myth not because their bodies have lost the ability to perform, but because they believe they have lost the ability to perform.	Sexually, men and women in good health can function effectively throughout their lives.
Alcohol ingestion reduces inhibitions and therefore enhances sexual enjoyment.	Many individuals use alcohol in the hope that it will increase their sexual pleasure and performance. Alcohol ingestion can also provide an excuse for engaging in sexual behaviors, e.g. "I would never have gone to bed with him if I hadn't had all that wine."	Data do not support the belief that alcohol ingestion reduces inhibitions and enhances sexual enjoyment.

Table 19-2   Nursing interventions in sexual responses of patients to nurses

Goal: Maintain a professional nurse-patient relationship that will enable nurse to provide therapeutic nursing care.

Principle	Rationale	Nursing Interventions
Establish a trusting relationship.	Atmosphere of trust allows for open, honest communication between patient and nurse; when this occurs, nurse can aid patient in discovering underlying issues related to patient's sexual feelings and behavior.	Express nonsexual caring and concern for patient. Be a responsible listener, especially to feelings and needs that patient may not be able to express directly. Reinforce purpose of professional, therapeutic nurse-patient relationship.
Be aware of own feelings and thoughts.	When aware of own feelings and thoughts, nurse will begin to understand how they influence behavior. With increased self-awareness, nurse increases effectiveness of interactions with patients.	Recognize own feelings and thoughts. Identify any specific patient interaction or behavior that influences feelings and thoughts. Identify influence of feelings and thoughts on behavior to increase effectiveness of interventions.

Continued

Table 19-2   Nursing interventions in sexual responses of patients to nurses—cont'd

Principle	Rationale	Nursing Interventions
Decrease patient's inappropriate expressions of sexual feelings and behavior.	If nurse can help patient see that the sexual interactions and behavior are being expressed to an inappropriate partner (nurse), sexual acting out will usually decrease. Nurse can help patient begin to identify reasons for behavior.	Set limits on patient's sexual behavior. Use a calm, matter-of-fact approach without implying judgment. Reaffirm nonsexual caring for patient. Explore meaning of patient's feelings and behavior.
Expand patient's insight into sexual feelings and behavior.	Once patient begins to identify reasons for sexual feelings and behaviors, patient can see that nurse is not an appropriate outlet for these feelings and behaviors. Patient then can move toward a more appropriate and therapeutic relationship with nurse.	Clarify misconceptions about any feeling patient may have about nurse as possible sexual partner. Point out futile nature of patient's romantic or sexual interest. Redirect patient's energies toward appropriate health-care issues.

Nursing Treatment Plan Summary
Maladaptive Sexual Responses

Nursing Diagnosis: Altered sexuality pattern
Expected Outcome: Patient will obtain the maximum level of adaptive sexual responses to enhance or maintain health.

Short-term Goals	Interventions	Rationale
Patient will describe values, beliefs, questions, and problems regarding sexuality.	Listen to sexual concerns implied and expressed.	An accepting therapeutic relationship will allow patients to be free to question, grow, and seek help with sexual concerns.
	Help patient explore sexual beliefs, values, and questions.	Communicate respect, acceptance, and openness to sexual concerns.
	Encourage open communication between patient and partner.	

Continued

Nursing Treatment Plan Summary
Maladaptive Sexual Responses—cont'd

Short-term Goals	Interventions	Rationale
Patient will relate accurate information about sexual concerns.	Clarify sexual misinformation. Dispel myths. Provide specific education about sexual health practices, behaviors, and problems. Give professional "permission" to continue sexual behavior that is not physically or emotionally harmful. Reinforce positive attitudes of patient.	Accurate information is helpful in changing negative thoughts and attitudes about particular aspects of sexuality. It can also prevent or limit dysfunctional behavior. Giving permission allows patient to continue the behavior and alleviate anxiety about normalcy. Patient can incorporate sexual behavior in a positive and accepting self-concept.

Patient will implement one new behavior to enhance sexual response.

Set clear goals with patient.

Identify specific behaviors that can be carried out, focusing on enhancing self-concept, role functioning, and sexuality.

Encourage relaxation techniques, redirection of attention, positional changes, and alternative ways of sexual expression as appropriate.

Become familiar with sexuality therapy resources available in the community.

Refer patient to a qualified sexuality therapist as needed.

Giving patient direct behavioral suggestions can help relieve a sexual problem or difficulty and is a useful intervention when the problem is of recent onset and short duration.

All nurses must screen for mal-adaptive sexual responses and provide basic nursing care, but should refer complex problems to qualified sexuality therapists for further treatment.

your **INTERNET**
c o n n e c t i o n

Healthy Sexuality
http://www.uiuc.edu/departments/mck...health-info/
sexual/intro/intro.htm
Homosexuality: Common Questions and
Statements Addressed
http://www.geocities.com/WestHollywood/1348/

Suggested readings

Augelli A, Patterson C: *Lesbian, gay and bisexual identities over the lifespan,* New York, 1995, Oxford University Press.

Beemer BR: Gender dysphoria update, *J Psychosoc Nurs* 34:13, 1996.

Butler R, Lewis M: *Love and sex after 60,* New York, 1993, Ballantine.

Cabaj R, Stein T: *Textbook of homosexuality and mental health,* Washington, DC, 1996, American Psychiatric Press.

Crenshaw TL, Goldberg JP: *Sexual pharmacology: drugs that affect sexual function,* New York, 1996, Norton.

Deevy S: Lesbian self-disclosure, *J Psychosoc Nurs* 31:21, 1993.

Fontaine K: Unlocking sexual issues: counseling strategies for nurses, *Nurs Clin North Am* 26:737, 1991.

Hellman R: Issues in the treatment of lesbian women and gay men with chronic mental illness, *Psychiatric Serv* 47:1093, 1996.

Kettl P et al: Sexual harassment of health care students by patients, *J Psychosoc Nurs Ment Health Serv* 31:11, 1993.

McConaghy N: *Sexual behavior: problems and management,* New York, 1993, Plenum.

Michael RT, Gagnon JH, Laumann EO, Kolata G: *Sex in America: a definitive survey,* Boston, 1994, Little, Brown.

Rowlands P: Schizophrenia and sexuality, *Sex Marital Ther* 10:1, 1995.

Smith G: Nursing care challenges: homosexual psychiatric patients, *J Psychosoc Nurs Ment Health Serv* 30:15, 1992.

Steiner J et al: Psychoeducation about sexual issues in an acute treatment setting, *Hosp Comm Psychiatry* 45:4, 1994.

Stuart G, Laraia M: *Principles and practice of psychiatric nursing,* ed 6, St Louis, 1998, Mosby.

Stewart R: Female circumcision: implications for North American nurses, *J Psychosoc Nurs* 35:35, 1997.

Zawid CS: *Sexual health: a nurse's guide,* Albany, NY, 1994, Delmar.

Psycho-pharmacology 20

Role of the Nurse

The nurse should be knowledgeable about the psychopharmaco-logical strategies available, but this information must be used as one part of a holistic approach to patient care. The nurse's role includes the following:

1. *Patient assessment.* This provides a baseline view of each patient.
2. *Coordination of treatment modalities.* This integrates the varied and often confusing drug treatments for patients.
3. *Administration of psychopharmacological agents.* This provides a professionally designed and individualized drug administration regimen.
4. *Monitoring drug effects.* This includes both desired effects and side effects that patients may experience.
5. *Patient education.* This enables patients to take their medicines safely and effectively.
6. *Drug maintenance program.* This is designed to support the patient in aftercare settings for extended periods.
7. *Participation in interdisciplinary clinical research drug trials.* The nurse is an essential member of the team that researches the drugs used to treat patients with psychiatric disorders.
8. *Prescriptive authority.* Some psychiatric nurses who are qualified by education and experience in accordance with their state practice act are able to prescribe pharmacological agents to treat the symptoms and improve the functional status of patients with psychiatric illness.

A s s e s s m e n t

Before initiation of psychopharmacological treatment, a thorough psychiatric evaluation must be completed, including the following:

1. Physical examination
2. Laboratory studies
3. Mental status evaluation
4. Medical and psychiatric history
5. Medication history
6. Family history

The Medication Assessment Tool presented in Box 20-1 can be used to take a drug history.

NURSE ALERT.   Concurrent use of drugs, or polypharmacy, can enhance a specific therapeutic action, can be necessary to treat concurrent illnesses, and can counteract unwanted effects of the first drug. Unfortunately, several problems are associated with concurrent drug use, including confusion over therapeutic efficacy and side effects and development of drug interactions. Table 20-1 lists some of the more common interactions of psychotropic drugs and other substances.

Antianxiety and Sedative-Hypnotic Drugs

Antianxiety and sedative-hypnotic drugs are divided into two categories: the benzodiazepines and the nonbenzodiazepines, which include several classes of drugs. The benzodiazepines are the most widely prescribed drugs in the world, and in the last 20 years they have almost entirely replaced the barbiturates in the treatment of anxiety and sleep disorders. Their popularity is related to their effectiveness and wide margin of safety.

Benzodiazepines

Mechanism of action

The benzodiazepines are thought to exert their antianxiety effects through their powerful potentiation of the inhibitory neurotransmitter gamma-aminobutyric acid (GABA):

Box 20-1   Medication Assessment Tool

Obtain the following information from the patient and
other available sources for each of the four categories of
drugs/substances taken by the patient.

I. Prescribed psychiatric medications ever taken
II. Prescribed nonpsychiatric medications taken in past
6 months or taken for major medical illnesses if
more than 6 months ago
III. Over-the-counter medications taken in past 6
months

The following apply to categories I, II, and III:

A. Name of drug
B. Reason taken
C. Dates started and stopped
D. Highest daily dose
E. Who prescribed it?
F. Was it effective?
G. Side effects or adverse reactions
H. Was it taken as directed?
I. If not, how was it taken?
J. History of drugs taken by first-degree
relatives
K. Drugs taken that were prescribed to others

IV. Alcohol, tobacco, caffeine, street drugs

A. Name of substance
B. Dates and schedule of use
C. Summary of effects
D. Adverse reactions and withdrawal symptoms
E. Attempts and treatments to discontinue drug
F. Impact of substance on:
1. Quality of life
2. Relationships/spouse/children
3. Occupation/education
4. Health/productivity
5. Self-image
6. Expense

Table 20-1   Interaction of psychotropic drugs with other substances

Psychotropic Category/Interacting Category	Possible Interactions
ANTIANXIETY AGENTS	
Benzodiazepines with:	
CNS depressants—alcohol, barbiturates, antipsychotics, antihistamines, cimetidine	Potential additive CNS effects, especially sedation and decreased daytime performance
SSRIs, disulfiram, estrogens	Increased benzodiazepine effects
Antacids, tobacco	Decreased benzodiazepine effects
Sedative-Hypnotics with:	
CNS depressants—alcohol, antihistamines, antidepressants, narcotics, antipsychotics	Enhancement of sedative effects; impairment of mental and physical performance; may result in lethargy, respiratory depression, coma, and death
Anticoagulants (oral)*	Decreased coumarin plasma levels and effect; monitor and adjust dose of coumarin
ANTIDEPRESSANTS	
TCAs with:	
MAOIs*	May cause hypertensive crisis
Alcohol, other CNS depressants	Additive CNS depression; decreased TCA effect
Antihypertensives*— guanethidine, methyldopa, clonidine	Antagonism of antihypertensive effect

Antipsychotics, antiparkinsonian drugs	Increased TCA effect; confusion, delirium, ileus
Anticholinergics	Additive anticholinergic effects
Antiarrhythmics—quinidine, procainamide, propranolol	Additive antiarrhythmic effects; myocardial depression
SSRIs*	Increased TCA serum level/toxicity through inhibition of cytochrome P-450 system
Anticonvulsants	Decreased TCA effect; seizures
Tobacco	Decreased TCA plasma levels
SSRIs with:	
Clomipramine, maprotiline, bupropion, clozapine	Increased risk of seizures
MAOIs*	Serotonin syndrome
Barbiturates, benzodiazepines, narcotics	Increased CNS depression
Carbamazepine	Neurotoxicity: nausea, vomiting, vertigo, tinnitus, ataxia, lethargy, blurred vision
MAOIs with:	
Many drugs and foods	Hypertensive crisis
MOOD STABILIZERS	
Lithium with:	
Diuretic,* marijuana	Increased lithium levels/toxicity
SSRIs	Lithium toxicity; enhanced therapeutic effect
Nonsteroidal antiinflammatory agents*	Increased lithium levels/toxicity
Antipsychotics	Increased CNS toxicity

*Potentially clinically significant.

Continued

Table 20-1 Interaction of psychotropic drugs with other substances—cont'd

Psychotropic Category/Interacting Category	Possible Interactions
MOOD STABILIZERS—cont'd	
Lithium with:—cont'd	
Tetracyclines	Lithium intoxication
Angiotensin converting enzyme inhibitors	Confusion, ataxia, dysarthria, tremor, electrocardiographic changes
Carbamazepine with:	
Lithium	Lithium intoxification; increased effect; inhibits lithium-induced polyuria
Haloperidol	Decreased effect of either drug
Calcium channel blockers	Neurotoxicity; dizziness, nausea, diplopia, headache
Valproate	Decreased valproate serum concentration
Cimetidine, erythromycin, isoniazid	Somnolence, lethargy, dizziness, blurred vision, ataxia, nausea

Valproate with:

SSRIs, erythromycin, cimetidine	Increased valproate serum concentrations

ANTIPSYCHOTICS WITH:

Antacids, tea, coffee, milk, fruit juice	Decreased phenothiazine effect
CNS depressants—narcotics, antianxiety drugs, alcohol, antihistamines, barbiturates	Additive CNS depression
Anticholinergic agents—levodopa*	Additive atropine-like side effects; increased antiparkin-sonian effects
SSRIs	Increased neuroleptic serum level; EPS

Clozapine with:

Carbamazepine*	Additive bone marrow suppression
Benzodiazepines*	Circulatory collapse; respiratory arrest
SSRIs*	Increased risk of seizures

CNS, Central nervous system; *SSRIs,* selective serotonin reuptake inhibitors; *TCAs,* tricyclic antidepressants; *MAOIs,* monoamine oxidase inhibitors; *EPS,* extrapyramidal symptoms.
*Potentially clinically significant.

Clinical use

The benzodiazpines are frequently the drug of choice in the management of anxiety, insomnia, and stress-related conditions. Most experts believe that treatment with benzodiazepines should be brief, during specific stress. With supervision, however, they are often given for extended periods (Table 20-2).

The major indications for benzodiazepine use follow:
1. Generalized anxiety disorder
2. Anxiety associated with depression
3. Sleep disorders
4. Anxiety associated with phobic disorders
5. Posttraumatic stress disorder
6. Alcohol and drug withdrawal
7. Anxiety associated with medical disease
8. Musculoskeletal relaxation
9. Seizure disorders
10. Preoperative anxiety

Adverse reactions and nursing considerations

The benzodiazepines have a very high therapeutic index; thus overdoses of these drugs alone almost never cause fatalities. Side effects are common, dose related, and almost always harmless. Table 20-3 summarizes these reactions and identifies nursing considerations.

NURSE ALERT. The benzodiazepines generally are not as strongly addictive as thought if their discontinuation is accomplished by gradual tapering, if they have been used for appropriate purposes, and if their use has not been complicated by the use of other substances, such as chronic use of barbiturates or alcohol. Watch particularly for the following:
1. Sedation
2. Ataxia
3. Irritability
4. Memory problems

Nonbenzodiazepines

The nonbenzodiazepines have been largely replaced by the benzodiazepines, although they are used occasionally (Table 20-4).

Table 20-2 Antianxiety and sedative hypnotic drugs: benzodiazepines

Chemical Class/Generic Name (Trade Name)	Active Metabolites	Half-life (hours)	Days to Steady State	Dose Equivalence (mg)	Usual Adult Dose (mg/day)	Preparations
Antianxiety drugs						
Alprazolam (Xanax)	Yes*	12-20	3	0.5	0.5-4	PO
Chlordiazepoxide (Librium)	Yes	12-100	1-3	10	15-100	PO, IM, IV
Clonazepam (Klonopin)	No	18-50	3-8	—	0.5-10	PO
Clorazepate (Tranxene)	Yes	30-100	5-16	7.5	7.5-60	PO
Diazepam (Valium)	Yes	20-90	4-8	5	2-40	PO, SR, IM, IV
Halazepam (Paxipam)	Yes	20-100	4	20	80-160	PO
Lorazepam (Ativan)	No	10-20	2-3	1	2-4	PO, IM, IV
Oxazepam (Serax)	No	5-15	1-2	15	15-90	PO
Prazepam (Centrax)	Yes	30-200	5-32	10	10-60	PO
Sedative-Hypnotic Drugs						
Estazolam (ProSom)	No	10-24	1-2	1	1-2	PO
Flurazepam (Dalmane)	Yes	30-100	4-8	15	15-60	PO
Temazepam (Restoril)	No	10-20	2-3	15	15-30	PO
Triazolam (Halcion)	No	1.5-4	1	0.25	0.25-0.5	PO

PO, Oral tablet or capsule; *IM*, intramuscular; *IV*, intravenous; *SR*, oral slow-release tablet.
*Not significant.

Table 20-3   Side effects and nursing considerations: benzodiazepines

Side Effects	Nursing Considerations*
Common	
Drowsiness, sedation	Activity helpful; caution patient when using machinery.
Ataxia, dizziness	Caution with activity; prevent falls.
Feelings of detachment	Discourage social isolation.
Increased irritability or hostility	Observe; support; be alert for disinhibition.
Anterograde amnesia	Patient unable to recall events that occur while taking drug.
Tolerance, dependency, rebound insomnia/anxiety	Short-term use; discontinue, using a slow taper.
Rare	
Nausea	Administer dose with meals; decrease dose.
Headache	Patient usually responds to mild analgesic.
Confusion	Decrease dose.
Gross psychomotor impairment	Dose related; decrease dose.
Depression	Decrease dose; antidepressant treatment.
Paradoxical rage reaction	Discontinue drug.

*Benzodiazepines contraindicated in patients with drug or alcohol abuse.

NURSE ALERT.   Use of most nonbenzodiazepines has numerous disadvantages, as follows:
1. Tolerance develops to the antianxiety effects of barbiturates.
2. They are more addictive.
3. They cause serious and even lethal withdrawal reactions.

Table 20-4 Antianxiety and sedative-hypnotic drugs: nonbenzodiazepines class

Chemical Class/Generic Name (Trade Name)	Usual Adult Dose (mg)
Barbiturates	
Amobarbital (Amytal)	100-200
Butabarbital (Butisol)	100-200
Pentobarbital (Nembutal)	100-200
Phenobarbital	100-200
Secobarbital (Seconal)	100-200
Propanediol	
Meprobamate (Equanil)	200-800
Acetylenic alcohol	
Ethychlorvynol (Placidyl)	500-1000
Chloral derivative	
Chloral hydrate (Noctec, Somnos)	500-2000
Antihistamines	
Diphenhydramine (Benadryl)	50
Hydroxyzine (Atarax)	100 tid
Beta-adrenergic blocker	
Propranolol (Inderal)	10 qid
Anxiolytic (antianxiety drug)	
Buspirone (BuSpar)	10-40
Imidazopyridine	
Zolpidem (Ambien)	10

tid, Three times a day; *qid,* four times a day.

4. They are dangerous in overdose and cause central nervous system (CNS) depression.
5. They have a variety of dangerous drug interactions.

Antidepressants

The types of antidepressant drugs are tricyclics (TCAs), monoamine oxidase inhibitors (MAOIs), selective serotonin reuptake inhibitors (SSRIs), and a group of other antidepressants not in the first three classes (Table 20-5). The primary clinical indication for the use of antidepressant drugs is major depressive illness. They are also useful in the treatment of panic disorder, other anxiety

Table 20-5   Antidepressant drugs

Chemical Class/ Generic Name (Trade Name)	Usual Adult Dose (mg/day)	Preparations
Tricyclics		
Tertiary (parent)		
Amitryptiline (Elavil)	50-300	PO, IM
Clomipramine (Anafranil)	50-250	PO
Doxepin (Adapin, Sinequan)	50-300	PO, L
Imipramine (Tofranil)	50-300	PO, IM
Trimipramine (Surmontil)	50-300	PO
Secondary (metabolite)		
Desipramine (Norpramin)	50-300	PO
Nortriptyline (Pamelor)	50-100	PO, L
Protriptyline (Vivactil)	15-60	PO
Monoamine Oxidase Inhibitors		
Isocarboxazid (Marplan)	30-70	PO
Phenelzine (Nardil)	45-90	PO
Tranylcypromine (Parnate)	20-60	PO
Selective Serotonin Reuptake Inhibitors		
Fluoxetine (Prozac)	20-80	PO
Fluvoxamine (Luvox)	50-250	PO
Paroxetine (Paxil)	20-50	PO
Sertraline (Zoloft)	25-200	PO
Other Antidepressants		
Amoxapine (Asendin)	50-600	PO
Bupropion (Wellbutrin)	50-600*	PO
Maprotiline (Ludiomil)	50-225*	PO
Mirtazapine (Remeron)	15-45	PO
Nefazodone (Serzone)	200-500	PO
Trazodone (Desyrel)	50-600	PO
Venlafaxine (Effexor)	25-375	PO

PO, Oral tablet or capsule; *IM*, intramuscular; *L*, oral liquid.
*Antidepressants with a ceiling dose because of dose-related seizures.

disorders, and enuresis in children. Preliminary research studies suggest they are useful for attention deficit disorders in children and for bulimia and narcolepsy.

Tricyclic Antidepressants

Mechanism of action

The TCAs appear to regulate the brain's use of the neurotransmitters norepinephrine and serotonin.

Clinical use

With an acceptable cardiac history and an electrocardiogram (ECG) within normal limits, particularly for people over 40 years old, TCAs are safe and effective in the treatment of acute and long-term depressive illnesses.

Adverse reactions and nursing considerations

The nurse should know the common side effects of the antidepressants and be aware of toxic effects and their treatment. These drugs cause sedation and anticholinergic side effects, such as dry mouth, blurred vision, constipation, urinary retention, orthostatic hypotension, temporary confusion, tachycardia, and photosensitivity. Most of these are common, short-term side effects and can be minimized with a decrease in dose. Toxic side effects include confusion, poor concentration, hallucinations, delirium, seizures, respiratory depression, tachycardia, bradycardia, and coma.

NURSE ALERT
1. Tricyclic antidepressants can be lethal in overdose.
2. They have a 3- to 4-week delay before therapeutic response.
3. They have no known long-term adverse effects.
4. Tolerance to therapeutic effects does not develop.
5. Persistent side effects can often be minimized by a small decrease in dose.
6. TCAs do not cause physical addiction or psychological dependence.
7. They do not cause euphoria; thus they have no abuse potential.
8. They can be conveniently given once a day.

Monoamine Oxidase Inhibitors

Mechanism of action

MAOIs block monoamine oxidase in the brain and the rest of the body. By blocking MAO in the brain, less norepinephrine is metabolized, thus increasing its availability in the synapse.

Clinical use

MAOIs are very effective antidepressant and antipanic drugs that have been underused and overly feared. Because of the potential for hypertensive crisis when tyramine-containing foods and certain medicine are taken concomitantly with these drugs, careful health teaching of a reliable patient is important. Box 20-2 outlines dietary restrictions with MAOI therapy.

Adverse reactions and nursing considerations

Side effects of MAOIs include lightheadedness, constipation, sexual dysfunction, muscle twitching, drowsiness, dry mouth, fluid retention, insomnia, urinary hesitancy, and weight gain. Box 20-3 lists signs and treatment of hypertensive crisis during MAOI therapy.

NURSE ALERT
1. MAOIs may be lethal in overdose.
2. Dietary restrictions must begin several days before taking the medication, be maintained while taking the medication, and be continued for 2 weeks after discontinuing therapy.
3. These drugs are nonaddicting.
4. Tolerance does not develop for therapeutic effects.
5. MAOIs decrease the body's ability to use vitamin B_6; thus supplements may be necessary.

Selective Serotonin Reuptake Inhibitors

Mechanism of action

The SSRIs inhibit the reuptake of serotonin at the presynaptic membrane. Thus these drugs promote the neurotransmission of serotonin in the brain. One of the newer antidepressants, venlafaxine,

Box 20-2   Dietary Restrictions: 1 Day Before, During, and 2-6 Weeks After MAOI Therapy

Food and Beverage to Avoid

Cheese, especially aged or matured
Fermented or aged protein (meat or fish)
Pickled or smoked fish
Chianti and vermouth wines, tap (draft) beer
Yeast or protein extracts
Fava or broad bean pods
Liver, sausages, pepperoni, Salami, canned ham
Spoiled or overripe fruit
Banana peel, sauerkraut

Food and Beverages to be Consumed in Moderation

Chocolate
Yogurt, sour cream, cottage and cream cheese
Clear spirits and white wine
Avacado, raspberries
New Zealand spinach
Soy sauce
Aspartame, monosodium glutamate

Drugs to Avoid

Most other antidepressant drugs
Other MAOIs
Nasal and sinus decongestants
Allergy and hay fever remedies
Narcotics, especially meperidine
Asthma remedies
Local anesthetics with epinephrine
Weight-reducing pills, pep pills, stimulants
Cocaine, amphetamines
Other medications without first checking with
   clinician

Medications that May Need Dose Decreased

Insulin and oral hypoglycemics
Oral anticoagulants
Thiazide diuretics
Anticholinergic agents
Muscle relaxants

Modified from Bernstein JG: *Handbook of drug therapy in psychiatry*, ed 3, St Louis, 1995, Mosby.

Box 20-3   Signs and Treatment of Hypertensive Crisis During MAOI Therapy

Warning Signs

Increased blood pressure, palpitations, frequent headaches

Symptoms of Hypertensive Crisis

Sudden elevation of blood pressure
Explosive headache, occipital that may radiate frontally
Head and face flushed and feel "full"
Palpitations, chest pain
Sweating, fever
Nausea, vomiting
Dilated pupils
Photophobia
Intracranial bleeding

Treatment

Hold next MAOI dose.
Do not have patient lie down (elevates blood pressure in head).
Administer intramuscular chlorpromazine, 100 mg; repeat if necessary (*mechanism of action:* blocks norepinephrine).
Administer intravenous phentolamine slowly in 5 mg doses (*mechanism of action:* binds with norepinephrine receptor sites, blocking norepinephrine).
Manage fever with external cooling techniques.
Evaluate diet, adherence to regimen, and education.

raises the levels of serotonin and norepinephrine. Thus it has a broad spectrum of activity and is called a *nonselective reuptake inhibitor.*

Clinical use

SSRIs not only represent a new approach to the treatment of depression and other disorders (e.g., panic disorder, obsessive-compulsive disorder), but also may provide a safer treatment option than other antidepressants because they are relatively safe in overdose. In addition, the SSRIs have a safer side effect profile than the TCAs and MAOIs.

Adverse reactions and nursing considerations

The SSRIs have antidepressant effects comparable to the other classes of antidepressant drugs but without significant anticholinergic, cardiovascular, and sedative side effects. The most common side effects include nausea, diarrhea, insomnia, dry mouth, nervousness, headache, sexual dysfunction, drowsiness, dizziness, and sweating. Most of these are short-term side effects and can be minimized by supportive measures, titrating the dose, or changing the medication schedule.

Mood-Stabilizing Drugs

Table 20-6 lists the three major mood-stabilizing drugs.

Lithium

Mechanism of action

Lithium is a naturally occurring salt, and the exact mechanism of action is not fully understood. Many neurotransmitter functions are altered.

Clinical use

Acute episodes of mania and hypomania and recurrent bipolar illness are the most common indications for lithium treatment. Other disorders with an affective component, such as recurrent unipolar depression, schizoaffective disorder, catatonia, rage reac-

Table 20-6   Mood-stabilizing drugs

Generic Name (Trade Name)	Usual Adult Dose (mg/day)	Preparations
Lithium (Eskalith, Lithobid, Lithonate)	900-1800	PO, L, SR
Valproate (Depakote)	750 mg/day- 60 mg/kg/day	PO, L, SR
Carbamazepine (Tegretol)	200-1600	PO, L, C

PO, Oral tablet or capsule; *L,* oral liquid; *SR,* oral slow-release tablet; *C,* chewable tablet.

tions, and alcoholism, are sometimes effectively treated with lithium, especially when they are periodic or cyclical.

Adverse reactions and nursing considerations

Patients can take lithium for many years. They must be taught the common causes for an increase in lithium level and ways to stabilize a therapeutic level (Box 20-4). Lithium side effects include fine hand tremor, fatigue, headache, mental dullness, lethargy, polyuria, polydipsia, gastric irritation, mild nausea, vomiting, diarrhea, acne, ECG changes, and weight gain.

Signs of lithium toxicity are related to lithium levels and include anorexia, nausea, vomiting, diarrhea, coarse hand tremor, twitching, lethargy, dysarthria, ataxia, fever, irregular vital signs, seizures, and coma.

Box 20-4   Lithium Levels

Common Causes for Increased Lithium Levels

1. Decreased sodium intake
2. Diuretic therapy
3. Decreased renal functioning
4. Fluid and electrolyte loss: sweating, diarrhea, dehydration
5. Medical illness
6. Overdose

Ways to Maintain Stable Lithium Levels

1. Stabilize dosing schedule by dividing doses or using sustained-release capsules.
2. Maintain adequate dietary sodium and fluid intake (2 to 3 quarts/day).
3. Replace fluid and electrolytes during exercise or gastrointestinal illness.
4. Monitor signs and symptoms of lithium side effects and toxicity.
5. If patients forget a dose, they may take it if they missed dosing time by 2 hours; if longer than 2 hours; if longer than 2 hours, skip that dose and take the next dose; never double-up doses.

Anticonvulsants

In the last two decades, several anticonvulsant drugs have been used successfully to treat bipolar illness. Carbamazepine (Tegretol) has a variety of effects in the brain that help to stabilize mood. Side effects include drowsiness, dizziness, ataxia, blurred vision, nausea, vomiting, and skin rash. A rare but serious problem is agranulocytosis; thus blood levels and complete blood counts are monitored frequently. Valproate (Depakote) is another anticonvulsant used in the treatment of bipolar illness. It is well tolerated in general, and side effects include anorexia, nausea, vomiting, diarrhea, tremor, sedation, ataxia, weight gain, and very rarely, pancreatitis and hepatic dysfunction, which necessitate regular laboratory studies.

NURSE ALERT
1. Lithium toxicity is a life-threatening emergency.
2. Blood levels must be monitored frequently.
3. Treatment failures may occur.
4. Lithium can also be combined with other antidepressants.
5. Patients need careful education about maintenance of lithium levels.
6. Lithium is sometimes used to augment the efficacy of other antidepressants.

Antipsychotic Drugs

Mechanism of action

Antipsychotic drugs are dopamine antagonists and block dopamine receptors in various pathways in the brain. Atypical antipsychotics also enhance the effectiveness of serotonin.

Clinical use

Table 20-7 lists the most frequently prescribed antipsychotic drugs. The chemical classes of the conventional, "typical" antipsychotic drugs are distinguished by the extent, type, and severity of side effects produced. Their overall clinical efficacy at equivalent doses is similar.

The newer, atypical antipsychotic drugs, such as clozapine, risperidone, and olanzapine, have clinical effects superior to other classes of antipsychotics with minimal acute extrapyramidal side effects.

Table 20-7   Antipsychotic drugs

Chemical Class/ Generic Name (Trade Name)	Dose Equivalence (mg)	Usual Adult Dose (mg/day)	Preparations
Typical Antipsychotics			
Phenothiazines			
Chlorpromazine (Thorazine)	100	100-2000	PO, IM, L
Fluphenazine (Prolixin)	4	30	PO, IM, L, L-A (every 2-4 weeks)
Mesoridazine (Serentil)	50	100-400	PO, IM, L
Perphenazine (Trilafon)	10	8-64	PO, IM, L
Thioridazine (Mellaril)	100	100-800*	PO, L
Trifluoperazine (Stelazine)	5	5-60	PO, IM, L
Thioxanthene			
Thiothixene (Navane)	5	5-60	PO, IM, L
Butyrophenone			
Haloperidol (Haldol)	4	2-100	PO, IM, L, L-A (every 4 weeks)
Dibenzoxazepine			
Loxapine (Loxitane)	10	30-250	PO, IM, L
Dihydroindolone			
Molindone (Moban)	10	10-225	PO, L
Atypical Antipsychotics			
Clozapine (Clozaril)	50	100-900	PO
Olanzapine (Zyprexa)	2	10	PO
Risperidone (Risperdal)	1	1-6	PO

PO, Oral tablet or capsule; *IM,* intramuscular; *L,* oral liquid, concentrate, suspension, or elixir; *LA,* long-acting injectable preparations.
*Upper limit to avoid retinopathy.

The major uses of antipsychotic drugs are to manage schizophrenia, organic brain syndrome with psychosis, the manic phase of manic-depressive illness, and severe depression with psychosis. They are also useful for patients with severe anxiety who abuse drugs or alcohol, because the benzodiazepines are contraindicated for them.

Adverse reactions and nursing considerations

The side effects of antipsychotic drugs are many and varied and demand much clinical attention from the nurse for optimum care. Some side effects are merely uncomfortable for the patient, and most are easily treated, but some are life threatening. The nurse should pay particular attention to the extrapyramidal symptoms or syndromes (EPS), both short term and long term. The most common drugs to treat short-term EPS follow:

1. Benztropine, 1 to 6 mg/day
2. Trihexyphenidyl, 1 to 10 mg/day
3. Diphenhydramine, 25 to 150 mg/day

The most serious adverse effect of clozapine is agranulocytosis, which occurs in approximately 1% to 2% of patients. Table 20-8 lists some of the more common side effects and nursing considerations.

NURSE ALERT

Guidelines for antipsychotic drug administration follow:

1. Individualized dosage requirements vary greatly.
2. After initial divided doses, patients can receive doses once a day.
3. Symptom improvement usually occurs in 2 or 3 days to 2 weeks. Optimum effects may take several months.
4. Some patients require a lifetime of continuous medication treatment.
5. Observation for tardive dyskinesia (long-term EPS) should be done about monthly during long-term treatment with conventional antipsychotics.
6. Good clinical care for patients taking clozapine includes weekly complete blood counts to monitor for decreased white cell count and Clozaril prescriptions given for 1 week at a time.

Table 20-8 Side effects and nursing considerations: antipsychotic drugs

Side Effects	Nursing Care and Teaching Considerations
Extrapyramidal symptoms (EPS)	General treatment principles:
	1. Tolerance usually develops by third month.
	2. Decrease dose of drug.
	3. Add a drug to treat EPS, then taper before 3 months of antipsychotic administration.
	4. Use a drug with a lower EPS profile.
	5. Provide patient education and support.
1. Acute dystonic reactions: oculogyric crisis, torticollis (wryneck)	Frightening, painful spasms of major muscle groups of neck, back, and eyes; more common in children and young males and with high-potency drugs.
	Medicate with drugs to treat EPS; have respiratory support available.
	Taper dose gradually when discontinuing antipsychotics to avoid withdrawal dyskinesia.
2. Akathisia	Patient cannot remain still; pacing, inner restlessness, and leg aches are relieved by movement.
	Rule out anxiety or agitation; medicate.
3. Parkinson's syndrome: akinesia, cogwheel rigidity, fine tremor	More common in males and elderly patients; tolerance may not develop.
	Medicate with amantadine, a DA agonist; patient must have good renal function.

4. Tardive dyskinesia (TD)	Can occur after use (usually long use) of conventional antipsychotics; stereotyped involuntary movements: tongue protrusion, lip smacking, chewing, blinking, grimacing, choreiform movements of limbs and trunk, foot tapping. Assess patient often; consider changing to atypical antipsychotic drug.
Neuroleptic malignant syndrome (NMS)	Potentially fatal, with fever, tachycardia, sweating, muscle rigidity, tremor, incontinence, stupor, leukocytosis, elevated creatinine phosphokinase, renal failure; more common with high-potency drugs and in dehydrated persons. Discontinue all drugs; provide supportive symptomatic care: hydration, renal dialysis, ventilation, and fever reduction as appropriate; can treat with dantrolene or bromocriptine; antipsychotic drugs can be cautiously reintroduced eventually.
Seizures	Occur in approximately 1% of patients taking antipsychotics; clozapine has a 5% seizure rate in patients taking 600–900 mg/day; may have to discontinue clozapine.
Other side effects	
1. Agranulocytosis	This is an emergency; it develops abruptly, with fever, malaise, ulcerative sore throat, and leukopenia. High incidence (1%–2%) is associated with clozapine; must do weekly complete blood counts and prescribe only 1 week of drug at a time; discontinue drug immediately; patient may need reverse isolation and antibiotics.
2. Photosensitivity	Use sunscreen and sunglasses; cover body with clothing.
3. Anticholinergic effects	Symptoms include constipation, dry mouth, blurred vision, orthostatic hypotension, tachycardia, urinary retention, nasal congestion. Decrease dose; use alternate drug.
4. Sedation, weight gain	Decrease dose; change drug; keep patient active; reduce calories.

your **INTERNET**
c o n n e c t i o n

Psychopharmacology and Drug References on
The Mental Health Net
http://www.cmhcsys.com/guide/pro22.htm#A
Psychopharmacology TIPS
http://uhs.bsd.uchicago.edu/~bhsiung/tips

Suggested readings

Benkert O et al: Public opinion on psychotropic drugs: an analysis of the factors influencing acceptance or rejection, *J Nervous Mental Dis* 3:151, 1997.

Bernstein JG: Drug interactions. In Bernstein JG, editor: *Handbook of drug therapy in psychiatry,* ed 3, St Louis, 1995, Mosby.

Brunello N, Langer SZ, Perez J, Racagni G: Current understanding of the mechanism of action of classic and newer antidepressant drugs, *Depression* 2:119, 1995.

Cornwell C, Chiverton P: The psychiatric advanced practice nurse with prescriptive authority: role development, practice issues, and outcomes measurement, *Arch Psychiatric Nurs* 2:57, 1997.

Crane K, Kirby B, Kooperman D: Patient compliance for psychotropic medications: a group model for an expanding psychiatric inpatient unit, *J Psychosoc Nurs* 34:8, 1996.

Glod CA, Mathieu J: Expanding uses of anticonvulsants in the treatment of bipolar disorder, *J Psychosoc Nurs Mental Health Serv* 31:37, 1993.

Jibson MD, Tandon R: A summary of research findings on the new antipsychotic drugs: special report, *Psychiatr Nurs Forum* 2, 1996.

Keltner N: Catastrophic consequences secondary to psychotropic drugs, *J Psychosoc Nurs* 35:41, Part I and Part II, 1997.

Lakshman M, Fernando D, Kazarian SS: Patient education in the drug treatment of psychiatric disorders: effect on compliance and outcome, *CNS Drugs* 3:291, 1995.

Lin KM, Poland RE, Nakasaki G: *Psychopharmacology and psychobiology of ethnicity,* Washington, DC, 1993, American Psychiatric Press.

Stuart G, Laraia M: *Principles and practice of psychiatric nursing,* ed 6, St Louis, 1998, Mosby.

Van Dongen CJ: Is the treatment worse than the cure? Attitudes toward medications among persons wtih severe mental illness, *J Psychosoc Nurs* 35:21, 1997.

Weiden PJ: How to evaluate for acute medication-induced movement disorders, *J Pract Psychiatry Behav Health* 2:176, 1996.

Weiden PJ: Prevention for acute extrapyramidal side effects, *J Pract Psychiatry Behav Health* 2:240, 1996.

Somatic Treatments

21

Many somatic treatments have been used in psychiatric settings. As research into the pathophysiology of mental illness continues, more and increasingly sophisticated somatic treatment modalities will likely be developed. At the same time, treatment modalities such as restraint, which was among the earliest means of providing nursing care for psychiatric patients, are still used. This chapter discusses the somatic therapies of mechanical restraints, seclusion, electroconvulsive therapy, and phototherapy.

Physical Restraints

Physical restraint includes the use of mechanical restraints, such as wrist or ankle cuffs and restraining sheets, as well as seclusion, which is confinement to a room from which the patient is unable to exit at will. In this era of sensitivity to civil liberties and individual rights, restraint should be used with great discretion.

Mechanical Restraints

Types of mechanical restraints are (1) camisoles (straitjackets), (2) wrist cuff restraints, (3) ankle cuff restraints, and (4) sheet restraints.

NURSE ALERT. *Prevention* of behavior necessitating restraints is the most important nursing action. Restraint is always an intervention of last resort.

Indications for Restraint

Indications for restraint are as follows:

1. Violent behavior that is dangerous to the patient or others
2. Agitated behavior that cannot be controlled by medication
3. Threat to physical integrity related to the patient's refusal to rest or eat and drink
4. Patient's request for external behavioral controls, provided this is assessed to be therapeutically indicated

Table 21-1 presents nursing interventions for restrained patients.

Cold Wet Sheet Packs

Patients can be immobilized by wrapping them in layers of sheets and blankets. The innermost layer consists of sheets that have been soaked in ice water. Although cold at first, the wrappings quickly become warm and soothing.

Use of this treatment modality is indicated by violent or agitated behavior that cannot be controlled by medication.

Nursing interventions include the following:

1. Place patient in a hospital gown on a bed with a waterproof mattress.
2. Wrap sheet snugly around the patient, taking care that no skin surfaces are in contact with each other.
3. Cover the wet sheets with a layer of blankets.
4. Observe the patient constantly.
5. Monitor temperature, pulse, and respirations. If any significant variation is noticed, discontinue the pack.
6. Offer fluids frequently.
7. Maintain restful environment.
8. Verbal contact should be quiet and soothing.
9. Discontinue pack after about 2 hours.
10. Provide skin care before assisting the patient to dress.

NURSE ALERT. Patients in any type of physical restraint are vulnerable and must be protected.

Seclusion

Seclusion is confinement in a room that the patient is unable to leave at will. Degrees of seclusion may range from confinement in

Table 21-1   Nursing interventions for a secluded or mechanically restrained patient

Principle	Rationale	Nursing Interventions
Patient has a right to least restrictive treatment.	This is a constitutional right of all patients.	Identify precipitating events. Observe patient for agitated behavior. Attempt alternative interventions. Document patient behavior and nursing interventions.
Protect patient from physical injury.	An individual who is not in control of behavior is at risk of injury and needs external limits, safely applied.	Provide adequate staff resources to control patient. Be sure staff is trained to manage violent behavior. Plan the approach to patient. Use safe physical restraint techniques.
Provide a safe environment.	An individual who is not in control of behavior may have impaired judgment and may harm self accidentally or purposefully.	Observe patient constantly or very frequently, depending on condition. Remove dangerous objects from area.

Continued

Table 21-1   Nursing interventions for a secluded or mechanically restrained patient—cont'd

Principle	Rationale	Nursing Interventions
Maintain biological integrity.	Physically restrained patients are not able to attend to their own biological needs and are at risk for complications related to immobility.	Check vital signs. Bathe patient and provide skin care. Take patient to bathroom or provide bedpan or urinal. Regulate room temperature. Position patient anatomically. Pad restraints. Offer food and fluids. Release restraints at least every 2 hours.
Maintain dignity and self-esteem.	Loss of control and imposition of physical restraint may be embarassing to patient.	Provide privacy. Explain situation to other patients without revealing confidential patient information. Maintain verbal contact with patient at regular intervals while awake. Assign consistent staff member of same sex to provide personal care. Involve patient in plans to terminate physical restraint. Wean patient from protected setting.

a room with a closed but unlocked door to a locked room with a mattress without linens on the floor, limited opportunity for communication, and the patient dressed in a hospital gown or a heavy canvas coverall. The latter are minimally acceptable conditions for seclusion and are used only when essential for the protection of the patient or others.

Indications for seclusion follow:

1. Control of violent behavior that is potentially dangerous to the patient or others and cannot be controlled by other less restrictive interventions such as interpersonal contact or medications
2. Reduction of environmental stimuli, particularly if requested by the patient

Contraindications include the following:

1. Need for observation for a medical problem
2. High suicide risk
3. Potential for intolerance of sensory deprivation
4. Punishment

Table 21-1 presents nursing interventions for secluded patients. Box 21-1 outlines the procedure for managing psychiatric emergencies.

Electroconvulsive Therapy

Electroconvulsive therapy (ECT) artificially induces a grand mal seizure by passing an electrical current through electrodes applied to one or both temples. The number of treatments given in a series varies according to the patient's initial problem and therapeutic response as assessed during treatment. The most common range for affective disorders is 6 to 12 treatments, whereas as many as 30 may be given for schizophrenia. ECT is usually administered three times a week on alternate days, although it can be given more or less frequently.

Indications for ECT follow:

1. Patients with major depressive illness who have not responded to antidepressant medication or who are unable to take medication
2. Patients with bipolar disorder who have not responded to medication
3. Acutely suicidal patients who have not received medication long enough to achieve a therapeutic effect

---

Box 21-1   Procedure for Managing Psychiatric Emergencies

---

1. Identify crisis leader.
2. Assemble crisis team.
3. Notify security officers if necessary.
4. Remove all other patients from area.
5. Obtain restraints if appropriate.
6. Devise a plan to manage crisis and inform team.
7. Assign securing of patient's limbs to crisis team members.
8. Explain necessity of intervention to patient and attempt to enlist cooperation.
9. Restrain patient when directed by crisis leader.
10. Administer medication if ordered.
11. Maintain calm, consistent approach to patient.
12. Review crisis management interventions with crisis team.
13. Process events with other patients and staff as appropriate.
14. Gradually reintegrate patient into milieu.

---

4. When the anticipated side effects of ECT are less than those associated with drug therapy, such as with elderly patients, for patients with heart block, and during pregnancy

The following is a summary of correct ECT procedure:

1. Provide patient and family education about the procedure.
2. Obtain informed consent.
3. Ensure NPO (nothing by mouth) status of the patient after midnight.
4. Ask the patient to remove jewelry, hairpins, eyeglasses, and hearing aids. Full dentures are removed; partial plates remain in place.
5. Dress the patient in loose, comfortable clothing.
6. Have the patient empty bladder.
7. Administer pretreatment medications.
8. Ensure necessary drugs and equipment are available and in working order (Box 21-2).

Box 21-2   Equipment for Electroconvulsive Therapy (ECT)

- Treatment device and supplies, including electrode paste and gel, gauze pads, alcohol preps, saline, electroencephalogram (EEG) electrodes, and chart paper
- Monitoring equipment, including electrocardiogram (ECG) and ECG electrodes
- Blood pressure cuffs (2), peripheral nerve stimulator, and pulse oximeter
- Stethoscope
- Reflex hammer
- Intravenous and venipuncture supplies
- Bite blocks with individual containers
- Stretcher with firm mattress and siderails and capability to elevate head and feet
- Suction device
- Ventilation equipment, including tubing, masks, Ambu bags, oral airways, and intubation equipment with an oxygen delivery system capable of providing positive-pressure oxygen
- Emergency and other medications as recommended by anesthesia staff
- Miscellaneous medications not supplied by the anesthesia staff for medical management during ECT, such as labetalol, esmolol, glycopyrrolate, caffeine, curare, midazolam, diazepam, thiopental sodium (Pentothal Sodium), methohexital sodium (Brevital Sodium), and succinylcholine

9. Assist with administration of ECT.
   - Reassure the patient.
   - The physician or anesthesiologist will administer oxygen to prepare the patient for the period of apnea that results from the muscle relaxant.
   - Administer medications.
   - Position padded mouth gag to protect the patient's teeth.
   - Position electrodes. The shock is then given.

10. Monitor the patient during the recovery period.
   - Assist as needed with the administration of oxygen and suctioning.
   - Monitor vital signs.
   - After respiration is established, position the patient on side until conscious. Maintain a patent airway.
   - When the patient is responsive, provide orientation.
   - Ambulate with assistance, after checking for postural hypotension.
   - Allow the patient to sleep for a short time if desired.
   - Provide a light meal.
   - Involve in usual daily activities, providing orientation as needed.
   - Offer prescribed analgesia for headache as necessary.

Table 21-2 summarizes nursing interventions for the patient receiving ECT.

Phototherapy

Phototherapy, or light therapy, consists of exposing patients to artificial therapeutic lighting about 5 to 20 times brighter than indoor lighting. Patients usually sit with eyes open, about 3 feet away from and at eye level with broad-spectrum fluorescent bulbs designed to produce the intensity and color composition of outdoor light. The timing and dosage of light therapy vary for each patient. The brighter the light, the more effective is the treatment per unit of time.

Effectiveness

Treatment is rapid and can be effective. Most patients feel relief after 3 to 5 days and relapse when treatment is stopped. Patients do not appear to develop tolerance to phototherapy, but its long-term efficacy has not been fully evaluated.

Indications

Phototherapy has a 50% to 60% response rate in patients with well-documented nonpsychotic winter depression or seasonal affective disorder (SAD). Light therapy should be administered by a professional with experience and training.

Table 21-2   Nursing interventions for a patient receiving electroconvulsive therapy (ECT)

Principle	Rationale	Nursing Interventions
Obtain informed participation in the procedure.	A patient who understands the treatment plan will be more cooperative and experience less stress than one who does not. An informed family is able to provide patient with emotional support.	Educate about ECT, including procedure and expected effects. Teach family about treatment. Encourage expression of feelings by patient and family. Reinforce teaching after each treatment.
Maintain biological integrity.	General anesthesia and an electrically induced seizure are physiological stressors and require supportive nursing care.	Check emergency equipment before procedure. Keep patient NPO several hours before treatment. Remove potentially harmful objects (e.g., jewelry, dentures). Check vital signs. Maintain patent airway. Position on side until reactive. Assist to ambulate. Offer analgesia or antiemetic as needed.
Maintain patient's dignity and self-esteem.	Patients are usually fearful before the treatment. Amnesia and confusion may led to fear of becoming insane. Patient will need assistance to function appropriately in the milieu.	Remain with patient and offer support before and during treatment. Maintain patient's privacy during and after treatment. Reorient patient. Assist family members and other patients to understand behavior related to amnesia and confusion.

your **INTERNET**
c o n n e c t i o n

Beyond Stigma: ECT and Depression
http://www.frii.com/~hageseth/index.html
Health Care Information Resources: Alternative
Medicine
http://www-hsl.mcmaster.ca/tomflem/altmed.html

Suggested readings

American Psychiatric Association Task Force on Clinician Safety: *Clinical safety (task force report 33),* Washington, DC, 1993, The Association.

Borum R, Swartz M, Swanson J: Assessing and managing violence risk in clinical practice, *J Pract Psychiatry Behav Health* 2:205, 1996.

Burns C, Stuart G: Nursing care in electroconvulsive therapy, *Psychiatr Clin North Am* 14:971, 1991.

Corrigan P, Yudofsky S, Silver J: Pharmacological and behavioral treatments for aggressive psychiatric inpatients, *Hosp Community Psychiatry* 44:125, 1993.

Fox H: Electroconvulsive therapy: an overview, *J Pract Psychiatry Behav Health* 2:223, 1996.

Harris D, Morrison E: Managing violence without coercion, *Arch Psychiatr Nurs* 9:203, 1995.

Kellner C, Pritchett J, Coffey C: *Handbook of ECT,* Washington, DC, 1997, American Psychiatric Press.

Martin K: Improving staff safety through an aggression management program, *Arch Psychiatr Nurs* 9:211, 1995.

McEnany G: Phototherapy & sleep manipulations: an examination of two nondrug biologic interventions for depression, *J Am Psychiatr Nurs Assoc* 2:86, 1996.

Morales E, Duphorne P: Least restrictive measures: alternatives to four-point restraints and seclusion, *J Psychosoc Nurs* 33:13, 1995.

Norris M, Kennedy C: How patients perceive the seclusion process, *J Psychosoc Nurs Ment Health Serv* 30:7, 1992.

Rosethal N: *Winter blues: SAD—what it is and how to overcome it,* New York, 1993, Guilford.

Stuart G, Laraia M: *Principles and practice of psychiatric nursing,* ed 6, St Louis, 1998, Mosby.

Tardiff K: *Concise guide to assessment and management of violent patients,* Washington, DC, 1996, American Psychiatric Press.

Tesar G: The agitated patient. Part I. Evaluation and behavioral management, *Hosp Community Psychiatry* 44:329, 1993.

Appendix A
Your Internet
Connection

Alzheimer's Association: http://www.alz.org/

American Association of Suicidology: http://www.cyberpsych.org/aas.htm

American Nurses Association: NURSINGWORLD: http://www.ana.org

American Psychiatric Nurses Association: http://www.apna.org

Anorexia Nervosa and Bulimia Association: http://qlink.queensu.ca/~4map/anabhome.htm

APA Online: American Psychiatric Association: http://www.psych.org/

Association of Managed Care Providers: http://www.comed.com/amcp

Bazelon Center for Mental Health Law: http://www.bazelon.org/

Beyond Stigma: ECT and Depression: http://www.frii.com/~hageseth

BPD CENTRAL: Borderline Personality Disorder Page: http://www.cmhc.com/disorders/sx10t.htm

Canadian Nurses Association: http://www.cna-nurses.ca/

Dual Diagnosis Website: http://www.erols.com/ksciacca/

Family Caregiver Alliance: http://www.caregiver.org/

Guide to Psychotherapy: http://www.shef.ac.uk/~psysc/psychotherapy

Guide to Psychotherapy: Self Esteem: http://www.shef.ac.uk/~psych/psychotherapy/esteem.htm/

Health Care Information Resources: Alternative Medicine: http://www-hsl.mcmaster.ca/tomflem/altmed.html

Healthy Sexuality: http://www.cyfernet.mes.umn.edu

Help! A Consumer's Guide to Mental Health Information: http://www.iComm.ca/madmagic/help/help.html

Homosexuality: Common Questions and Statements Addressed: http://www.geocities.com/WestHollywood/1348/

Institute for Behavior Health Care: http://www.ibh.com

Internet Depression Resources List: http://www.execpc.com/~corbeau/

Internet Mental Health: http://www.mentalhealth.com/

Life Sciences Institute of Mind—Body Health Presents: Self-Regulation of Mind & Body: http://www.cjnetworks.com/~lifesci/

Mental Health Net: http://www.cmhcsys.com

Multiple Personality & Dissociative Disorders: http://members.tripod.com/~fsrvival/

NAMI: National Alliance for the Mentally Ill: http://www.nami.org/

NAPD News: National Panic/Anxiety Disorder News: http://www.npadnews.com

NARSAD: National Alliance for Research on Schizophrenia and Depression: http://www.mhsource.com/narsad.html

National Institute of Mental Health: http://www.nimh.nih.gov

Neurosciences on the Internet: http://www.lm.com/~nab

Noodles' Panic—Anxiety Page: The ANXIETY—Panic Internet Resource: http://www.algy.com/anxiety

NursingNet: http://www.nursingnet.org/

Pendulum's Bipolar Disorder/Manic-Depression Page: http://www.pendulum.org/

Psychopharmacology and Drug References on the Mental Health Net: http://www.cmhcsys.com/guide/pro22.htm#A

Psychopharmacology TIPS: http://uhs.bsd.uchicago.edu/~bhsiung/tips

The Schizophrenia Home Page: http://www.schizophrenia.com/

The SLEEP WELL: http://www-leland.stanford.edu/~dement/

The Something Fishy Website on Eating Disorders: http://www.something-fishy.com/edsa.htm

Suicide Awareness/Voices of Education (SAVE): http://www.save.org/

WEB of Addictions: http://www.well.com/user/woa/

Index

NOTES

NANDA Diagnoses

Activity intolerance
Activity intolerance, risk for
Adaptive capacity: intracranial, decreased
Adjustment, impaired
Airway clearance, ineffective
Alcoholism, altered family process
Anxiety
Aspiration, risk for
Body image disturbance
Body temperature, altered, risk for
Bowel incontinence
Breastfeeding, effective
Breastfeeding, ineffective
Breastfeeding, interrupted,
Breathing pattern, ineffective
Cardiac output, decreased
Caregiver role strain
Caregiver role strain, risk for
Communication, impaired verbal
Community coping, potential for enhanced
Community coping, ineffective
Confusion, acute
Confusion, chronic
Constipation
Constipation, colonic
Constipation, perceived
Coping, defensive
Coping, family, potential for growth
Coping, ineffective family: compromised
Coping, ineffective family: disabling
Coping, ineffective individual
Decisional conflict (specify)
Denial, ineffective
Diarrhea
Disuse syndrome, risk for

Diversional activity deficit
Dysreflexia
Energy field disturbance
Environmental interpretation syndrome, impaired
Family processes, altered: alcoholism
Family processed, altered
Fatigue
Fear
Fluid volume deficit
Fluid volume deficit, risk for
Fluid volume excess
Gas exchange, impaired
Grieving, anticipatory
Grieving, dysfunctional
Growth and development, altered
Health maintenance, altered
Health-seeking behaviors (specify)
Home maintenance management, impaired
Hopelessness
Hyperthermia
Hypothermia
Incontinence, functional
Incontinence, reflex
Incontinence, stress
Incontinence, total
Incontinence, urge
Infant behavior, disorganized
Infant behavior, disorganized: risk for
Infant behavior, organized, potential for enhanced
Infant feeding pattern, ineffective
Infection, risk for
Injury, perioperative positioning: risk for
Injury, risk for